TRAUMATIC BRAIN INJURY
SOURCEBOOK
FIRST EDITION

Health Reference Series

TRAUMATIC BRAIN INJURY
SOURCEBOOK

FIRST EDITION

Basic Consumer Health Information about Traumatic Brain Injury (TBI), Its Symptoms, Diagnosis, and Treatments Including Facts about Disabilities and Other Conditions Associated with TBI, and Safety Measures

Along with Information on Rehabilitation Techniques, Caring for People Affected with TBI, a Glossary of Terms, and a Directory of Organizations for Additional Help and Information

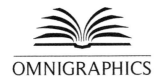

OMNIGRAPHICS

615 Griswold St., Ste. 520, Detroit, MI 48226

Bibliographic Note

Because this page cannot legibly accommodate all the copyright notices,
the Bibliographic Note portion of the Preface constitutes an extension
of the copyright notice.

* * *

OMNIGRAPHICS
Kevin Hayes, *Managing Editor*

* * *

Library of Congress Cataloging-in-Publication Data

Names: Omnigraphics, Inc., issuing body.

Title: Traumatic brain injury sourcebook: basic consumer health information about traumatic brain injury (TBI), its symptoms, diagnosis, and treatments including disabilities and other conditions associated with TBI, and coping with TBI along with information on rehabilitation techniques, caring for people affected with TBI, a glossary of terms, and a directory of organizations for additional help and Information.

Description: First edition. | Detroit: Omnigraphics, Inc., 2020. | Series: Health reference series | Includes index. | Summary: "Provides primary health information on traumatic brain injury (TBI), its symptoms, diagnosis, and treatments, other conditions and disabilities that occur due to TBI, and coping methods. Includes a glossary of terms and directory of organizations for additional help and information"-- Provided by publisher.

Identifiers: LCCN 2020007940 (print) | LCCN 2020007941 (ebook) | ISBN 9780780818002 (library binding) | ISBN 9780780818019 (ebook)

Subjects: LCSH: Brain damage. | Brain damage--Diagnosis. | Brain damage--Treatment.

Classification: LCC RC387.5.T748 2020 (print) | LCC RC387.5 (ebook) | DDC 617.4/81--dc23

LC record available at https://lccn.loc.gov/2020007940
LC ebook record available at https://lccn.loc.gov/2020007941

Table of Contents

Part 5. Reducing the Risk of Traumatic Brain Injury

Part 6. Living with Traumatic Brain Injury

Part 7. Clinical Trials and Research Studies on Traumatic Brain Injury

Preface

ABOUT THIS BOOK

Traumatic brain injury (TBI) occurs when there is a sudden trauma that results in damage to the brain. This can occur when a person's head violently hits an object or when an object pierces the skull and enters brain tissue. It may occur even without a direct blow to the head, such as when a person suffers a whiplash. Depending on the extent of damage to the brain, the symptoms of TBI can be mild, moderate, or severe. According to the Centers for Disease Control and Prevention (CDC), in 2014, there were about 2.87 million TBI-related emergency department (ED) visits, hospitalizations, and deaths in the United States including 837,000 children.

Traumatic Brain Injury Sourcebook, First Edition begins with basics of the brain. It provides information and facts about traumatic brain injury along with its classifications, symptoms, and potential effects. It offers information on diagnosis, treatment, and surgical options of TBI. It discusses various conditions associated with TBI, such as Alzheimer disease, dementia, Parkinson disease, etc., and deals with the disabilities that may occur as a result of TBI. It talks about various safety measures to be taken to avoid a brain injury. Rehabilitation techniques and caring for those affected with TBI are discussed. Facts about some important clinical trials and research studies on TBI are also provided. The book concludes with a glossary of terms related to traumatic brain injuries and resources for additional help and information.

HOW TO USE THIS BOOK

This book is divided into parts and chapters. Parts focus on broad areas of interest. Chapters are devoted to single topics within a part.

Part 1: Understanding Traumatic Brain Injury begins with a basic description of what the brain is and explains how it functions. It provides information and facts about traumatic brain injury (TBI) along with its classifications, symptoms, and potential effects. It also provides facts about high-risk groups for brain injury.

Part 2: Diagnosis and Treatment of Traumatic Brain Injury provides suggestions on when to seek medical help and what to expect from a healthcare professional. It offers information on diagnosis, treatment, and surgical options for TBI. Emergency treatment guidelines to help people with a severe brain injury are also provided.

Part 3: Conditions Associated with Traumatic Brain Injury talks about the various conditions associated with TBI such as Alzheimer disease, dementia, hypertension, Parkinson disease, posttraumatic stress disorder (PTSD), vision loss, and epilepsy.

Part 4: Disability from Traumatic Brain Injury offers information about severe disabilities resulting from a TBI. It talks about what disability is and explains how to live with a physical disability. It gives an insight into how people with a TBI or other disabilities are being victimized and offers information on how to seek support services.

Part 5: Reducing the Risk of Traumatic Brain Injury provides preventive measures to be taken to stay away from a brain injury. It talks about road safety, workplace safety, playground safety, and sports safety. It highlights the importance of helmets and explains how to use them properly.

Part 6: Living with Traumatic Brain Injury talks about rehabilitation and life after TBI. It explains how to manage specific symptoms caused by TBI and gives information about the role of parents in helping children with TBI. Some useful information on how to care for a person with TBI is also provided.

Part 7: Clinical Trials and Research Studies on Traumatic Brain Injury has basic information on what clinical trials and observational studies are, followed by information on some important clinical trials on TBI.

Part 8: Additional Help and Information provides a glossary of terms related to TBI and lists out the government and private organizations that provide help and support to people with TBI.

BIBLIOGRAPHIC NOTE

This volume contains documents and excerpts from publications issued by the following U.S. government agencies: Administration for Community

Living (ACL); Agency for Healthcare Research and Quality (AHRQ); Centers for Disease Control and Prevention (CDC); Child Welfare Information Gateway (CWIG); *Eunice Kennedy Shriver* National Institute of Child Health and Human Development (NICHD); National Center for Posttraumatic Stress Disorder (NCPTSD); National Highway Traffic Safety Administration (NHTSA); National Institute of Neurological Disorders and Stroke (NINDS); National Institute on Aging (NIA); National Institute on Drug Abuse (NIDA) for Teens; National Institutes of Health (NIH); Occupational Safety and Health Administration (OSHA); U.S. Consumer Product Safety Commission (CPSC); U.S. Department of Veterans Affairs (VA); U.S. Food and Drug Administration (FDA); and USA.gov.

It may also contain original material produced by Omnigraphics and reviewed by medical consultants.

ABOUT THE *HEALTH REFERENCE SERIES*

The *Health Reference Series* is designed to provide basic medical information for patients, families, caregivers, and the general public. Each volume provides comprehensive coverage on a particular topic. This is especially important for people who may be dealing with a newly diagnosed disease or a chronic disorder in themselves or in a family member. People looking for preventive guidance, information about disease warning signs, medical statistics, and risk factors for health problems will also find answers to their questions in the *Health Reference Series*. The *Series*, however, is not intended to serve as a tool for diagnosing illness, in prescribing treatments, or as a substitute for the physician–patient relationship. All people concerned about medical symptoms or the possibility of disease are encouraged to seek professional care from an appropriate healthcare provider.

A NOTE ABOUT SPELLING AND STYLE

Health Reference Series editors use *Stedman's Medical Dictionary* as an authority for questions related to the spelling of medical terms and *The Chicago Manual of Style* for questions related to grammatical structures, punctuation, and other editorial concerns. Consistent adherence is not always possible, however, because the individual volumes within the *Series* include many documents from a wide variety of different producers, and the editor's primary goal is to present material from each source as accurately as is possible. This sometimes means that information in different chapters or sections may follow other guidelines and alternate spelling authorities.

For example, occasionally a copyright holder may require that eponymous terms be shown in possessive forms (Crohn's disease vs. Crohn disease) or that British spelling norms be retained (leukaemia vs. leukemia).

MEDICAL REVIEW

Omnigraphics contracts with a team of qualified, senior medical professionals who serve as medical consultants for the *Health Reference Series*. As necessary, medical consultants review reprinted and originally written material for currency and accuracy. Citations including the phrase "Reviewed (month, year)" indicate material reviewed by this team. Medical consultation services are provided to the *Health Reference Series* editors by:

Dr. Vijayalakshmi, MBBS, DGO, MD
Dr. Senthil Selvan, MBBS, DCH, MD
Dr. K. Sivanandham, MBBS, DCH, MS (Research), PhD

OUR ADVISORY BOARD

We would like to thank the following board members for providing initial guidance on the development of this series:

- Dr. Lynda Baker, Associate Professor of Library and Information Science, Wayne State University, Detroit, MI
- Nancy Bulgarelli, William Beaumont Hospital Library, Royal Oak, MI
- Karen Imarisio, Bloomfield Township Public Library, Bloomfield Township, MI
- Karen Morgan, Mardigian Library, University of Michigan-Dearborn, Dearborn, MI
- Rosemary Orlando, St. Clair Shores Public Library, St. Clair Shores, MI

HEALTH REFERENCE SERIES UPDATE POLICY

The inaugural book in the *Health Reference Series* was the first edition of *Cancer Sourcebook* published in 1989. Since then, the *Series* has been enthusiastically received by librarians and in the medical community. In order to maintain the standard of providing high-quality health information for the layperson the editorial staff at Omnigraphics felt it was necessary to implement a policy of updating volumes when warranted.

Medical researchers have been making tremendous strides, and it is the purpose of the *Health Reference Series* to stay current with the most recent advances. Each decision to update a volume is made on an individual basis.

Some of the considerations include how much new information is available and the feedback we receive from people who use the books. If there is a topic you would like to see added to the update list, or an area of medical concern you feel has not been adequately addressed, please write to:

Managing Editor
Health Reference Series
Omnigraphics
615 Griswold St., Ste. 520
Detroit, MI 48226

Part 1 | **Understanding Traumatic Brain Injury**

Chapter 1 | Brain Basics: Know Your Brain

The brain is the most complex part of the human body. This three-pound organ is the seat of intelligence, interpreter of the senses, initiator of body movement, and controller of behavior. Lying in its bony shell and washed by protective fluid, the brain is the source of all the qualities that define humanity. The brain is the crown jewel of the human body.

For centuries, scientists and philosophers have been fascinated by the brain, but until recently they viewed the brain as nearly incomprehensible. Now, however, the brain is beginning to relinquish its secrets. Scientists have learned more about the brain in the last 10 years than in all previous centuries because of the accelerating pace of research in neurological and behavioral science and the development of new research techniques. As a result, Congress named the 1990s the Decade of the Brain. At the forefront of research on the brain and other elements of the nervous system is the National Institute of Neurological Disorders and Stroke (NINDS), which conducts and supports scientific studies in the United States and around the world.

THE ARCHITECTURE OF THE BRAIN

The brain is like a committee of experts. All the parts of the brain work together, but each part has its own special properties. The brain can be divided into three basic units: the forebrain, the midbrain, and the hindbrain.

This chapter includes text excerpted from "Brain Basics: Know Your Brain," National Institute of Neurological Disorders and Stroke (NINDS), February 13, 2020.

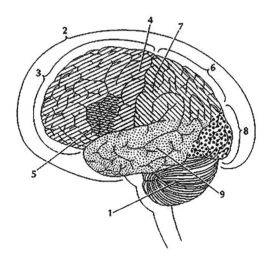

Figure 1.1. Know Your Brain

The hindbrain includes the upper part of the spinal cord, the brain stem, and a wrinkled ball of tissue called the "cerebellum" (1). The hindbrain controls the body's vital functions, such as respiration and heart rate. The cerebellum coordinates movement and is involved in learned rote movements. When you play the piano or hit a tennis ball you are activating the cerebellum. The uppermost part of the brainstem is the midbrain, which controls some reflex actions and is part of the circuit involved in the control of eye movements and other voluntary movements. The forebrain is the largest and most highly developed part of the human brain, it consists primarily of the cerebrum (2) and the structures hidden beneath it.

When people see pictures of the brain it is usually the cerebrum that they notice. The cerebrum sits at the topmost part of the brain and is the source of intellectual activities. It holds your memories, allows you to plan, enables you to imagine and think. It allows you to recognize friends, read books, and play games.

The cerebrum is split into two halves (hemispheres) by a deep fissure. Despite the split, the two cerebral hemispheres communicate with each other through a thick tract of nerve fibers that lies at the base of this fissure. Although the two hemispheres seem to

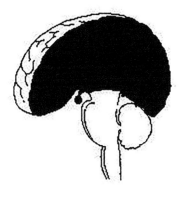 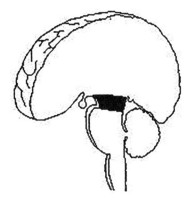

Figure 1.2. Forebrain   **Figure 1.3.** Midbrain

be mirror images of each other, they are different. For instance, the ability to form words seems to lie primarily in the left hemisphere, while the right hemisphere seems to control many abstract reasoning skills.

For some as-yet-unknown reason, nearly all of the signals from the brain to the body and vice-versa cross over on their way to and from the brain. This means that the right cerebral hemisphere primarily controls the left side of the body and the left hemisphere primarily controls the right side. When one side of the brain is damaged, the opposite side of the body is affected. For example, a stroke in the right hemisphere of the brain can leave the left arm and leg paralyzed.

THE GEOGRAPHY OF THOUGHT

Each cerebral hemisphere can be divided into sections, or lobes, each of which specializes in different functions. To understand each lobe and its specialty we will take a tour of the cerebral hemispheres, starting with the two frontal lobes (3), which lie directly behind the forehead. When you plan a schedule, imagine the future, or use reasoned arguments, these two lobes do much of the work. One of the ways the frontal lobes seem to do these things is by acting as short-term storage sites, allowing one idea to be kept in mind while other ideas are considered. In the rearmost portion of each frontal lobe, there is a motor area (4), which helps

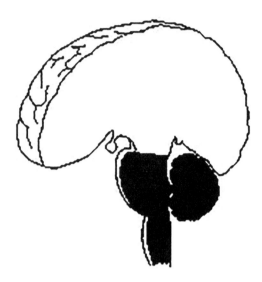

Figure 1.4. Hindbrain

control voluntary movement. A nearby place on the left frontal lobe called "Broca's area (5)" allows thoughts to be transformed into words.

When you enjoy a good meal—the taste, aroma, and texture of the food—two sections behind the frontal lobes called the "parietal lobes" (6) are at work. The forward parts of these lobes, just behind the motor areas, are the primary sensory areas (7). These areas receive information about temperature, taste, touch, and movement from the rest of the body. Reading and arithmetic are also functions in the repertoire of each parietal lobe.

Two areas at the back of the brain are at work, these lobes are called the "occipital lobes" (8), process images from the eyes and link that information with images stored in memory. Damage to the occipital lobes can cause blindness.

The last lobes of the cerebral hemispheres are the temporal lobes (9), which lie in front of the visual areas and nest under the parietal and frontal lobes. Whether you appreciate symphonies or rock music, your brain responds through the activity of these lobes. At the top of each temporal lobe is an area responsible for receiving information from the ears. The underside of each temporal lobe plays a crucial role in forming and retrieving memories, including those associated with music. Other parts of this lobe seem to integrate memories and sensations of taste, sound, sight, and touch.

THE CEREBRAL CORTEX

Coating the surface of the cerebrum and the cerebellum is a vital layer of tissue—the thickness of a stack of two or three dimes. It is called the "cortex," derived from the Latin word for bark. Most of the actual information processing in the brain takes place in the cerebral cortex. When people talk about "gray matter" in the brain they are talking about this thin rind. The cortex is gray because nerves in this area lack the insulation that makes most other parts of the brain appear to be white. The folds in the brain add to its surface area and, therefore, increase the amount of gray matter and the quantity of information that can be processed.

THE INNER BRAIN

Deep within the brain, hidden from view, lie structures that are the gatekeepers between the spinal cord and the cerebral hemispheres. These structures not only determine a person's emotional state, but also modifies their perceptions and responses depending on that state, and allow them to initiate movements that you make without thinking about them. Like the lobes in the cerebral hemispheres, the structures described below come in pairs: each is duplicated in the opposite half of the brain.

The hypothalamus (10), about the size of a pearl, directs a multitude of important functions. It wakes you up in the morning and gets the adrenaline flowing during a test or job interview. The hypothalamus is also an important emotional center, controlling the molecules that make you feel exhilarated, angry, or unhappy. Near the hypothalamus lies the thalamus (11), a major clearinghouse for information going to and from the spinal cord and the cerebrum.

An arching tract of nerve cells leads from the hypothalamus and the thalamus to the hippocampus (12). This tiny nub acts as a

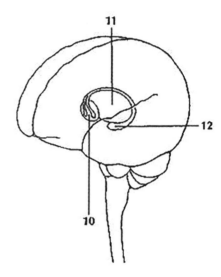

Figure 1.5. The Innerbrain

memory indexer—sending memories out to the appropriate part of the cerebral hemisphere for long-term storage and retrieving them when necessary. The basal ganglia are clusters of nerve cells surrounding the thalamus. They are responsible for initiating and integrating movements. Parkinson disease (PD)—which results in tremors, rigidity, and a stiff, shuffling walk—is a disease of nerve cells that lead into, the basal ganglia.

MAKING CONNECTIONS

The brain and the rest of the nervous system are composed of many different types of cells, but the primary functional unit is a cell called the "neuron." All sensations, movements, thoughts, memories, and feelings are the result of signals that pass through neurons. Neurons consist of three parts. The cell body (13) contains the nucleus, where most of the molecules that the neuron needs to survive and function are manufactured. Dendrites (14) extend out from the cell body like the branches of a tree and receive messages from other nerve cells. Signals then pass from the dendrites through the cell body and may travel away from the cell body down

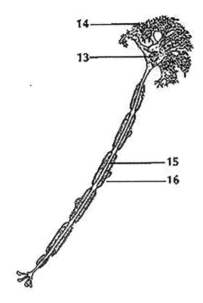

Figure 1.6. Making Connection

an axon (15) to another neuron, a muscle cell, or cells in some other organ. The neuron is usually surrounded by many support cells. Some types of cells wrap around the axon to form an insulating sheath (16). This sheath can include a fatty molecule called "myelin," which provides insulation for the axon and helps nerve signals travel faster and farther. Axons may be very short, such as those that carry signals from one cell in the cortex to another cell less than a hair's width away. Or axons may be very long, such as those that carry messages from the brain all the way down the spinal cord.

Scientists have learned a great deal about neurons by studying the synapse—the place where a signal passes from the neuron to another cell. When the signal reaches the end of the axon it stimulates the release of tiny sacs (17). These sacs release chemicals, known as, "neurotransmitters" (18) into the synapse (19). The neurotransmitters cross the synapse and attach to receptors (20) on the neighboring cell. These receptors can change the properties of the receiving cell. If the receiving cell is also a neuron, the signal can continue the transmission to the next cell.

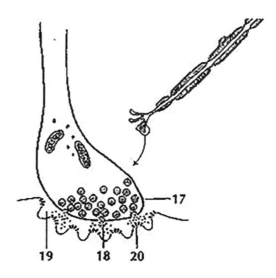

Figure 1.7. Cell Body

SOME KEY NEUROTRANSMITTERS AT WORK

Acetylcholine is called an "excitatory neurotransmitter" because it generally makes cells more excitable. It governs muscle contractions and causes glands to secrete hormones. Alzheimer disease (AD), which initially affects memory formation, is associated with a shortage of acetylcholine.

Gamma-aminobutyric acid (GABA) is called an "inhibitory neurotransmitter" because it tends to make cells less excitable. It helps control muscle activity and is an important part of the visual system. Drugs that increase GABA levels in the brain are used to treat epileptic seizures and tremors in patients with Huntington disease (HD).

Serotonin is a neurotransmitter that constricts blood vessels and brings on sleep. It is also involved in temperature regulation. Dopamine is an inhibitory neurotransmitter involved in the control of mood and complex movements. The loss of dopamine activity in some portions of the brain leads to the muscular rigidity of Parkinson disease (PD). Many medications used to treat behavioral disorders work by modifying the action of dopamine in the brain.

NEUROLOGICAL DISORDERS

When the brain is healthy it functions quickly and automatically. But, when problems occur, the results can be devastating. Some 50 million people in the United States—one in five—suffer from damage to the nervous system. The NINDS supports research on more than 600 neurological diseases. Some of the major types of disorders include:

- Neurogenetic diseases (such as Huntington disease and muscular dystrophy)
- Developmental disorders (such as cerebral palsy)
- Degenerative diseases of adult life (such as Parkinson disease and Alzheimer disease)
- Metabolic diseases (such as Gaucher disease)
- Cerebrovascular diseases (such as stroke and vascular dementia)
- Trauma (such as spinal cord and head injury)
- Convulsive disorders (such as epilepsy)
- Infectious diseases (such as acquired immunodeficiency syndrome (AIDS) dementia)
- Brain tumors

Chapter 2 | Overview of Traumatic Brain Injury

Chapter Contents

Section 2.1 | Traumatic Brain Injury: Basics

This section includes text excerpted from "Traumatic Brain Injury: Hope through Research," National Institute of Neurological Disorders and Stroke (NINDS), April 24, 2020.

WHAT IS A TRAUMATIC BRAIN INJURY?

A traumatic brain injury (TBI) can be caused by a forceful bump, blow, or jolt to the head or body, or from an object that pierces the skull and enters the brain. Not all blows or jolts to the head result in a TBI.

Some types of TBI can cause temporary or short-term problems with normal brain function, including problems with how the person thinks, understands, moves, communicates, and acts. More serious TBI can lead to severe and permanent disability, and even death.

Some injuries are considered primary, meaning the damage is immediate. Other outcomes of TBI can be secondary, meaning they can occur gradually over the course of hours, days, or appear weeks later. These secondary brain injuries are the result of reactive processes that occur after the initial head trauma. There are two broad types of head injuries: penetrating and nonpenetrating.

- Penetrating TBI (also known as "open TBI") happens when an object pierces the skull (for example, a bullet, shrapnel, bone fragment, or by a weapon, such as hammer or knife) and enters the brain tissue. Penetrating TBI typically damages only part of the brain.
- Nonpenetrating TBI (also known as "closed head injury" or "blunt TBI") is caused by an external force strong enough to move the brain within the skull. Causes include falls, motor vehicle crashes, sports injuries, blast injury, or being struck by an object.

Some accidents such as explosions, natural disasters, or other extreme events can cause both penetrating and nonpenetrating TBI in the same person.

WHAT ARE THE SIGNS AND SYMPTOMS OF TRAUMATIC BRAIN INJURY?

Seek immediate medical attention if you experience any of the following physical, cognitive/behavioral, or sensory symptoms, especially within the first 24 hours after a TBI:

- **Physical**
  - Headache
  - Convulsions or seizures
  - Blurred or double vision
  - Unequal eye pupil size or dilation
  - Clear fluids draining from the nose or ears
  - Nausea and vomiting
  - New neurologic deficit, i.e., slurred speech; weakness of arms, legs, or face; loss of balance
- **Cognitive/Behavioral**
  - Loss of or change in consciousness anywhere from a few seconds to a few hours
  - Decreased level of consciousness, i.e., hard to awaken
  - Mild to profound confusion or disorientation
  - Problems remembering, concentrating, or making decisions
  - Changes in sleep patterns (e.g., sleeping more, difficulty falling or staying asleep); inability to waken from sleep
  - Frustration, irritability
- **Perception/sensation**
  - Light-headedness, dizziness, vertigo, or loss of balance or coordination
  - Blurred vision
  - Hearing problems, such as ringing in the ears
  - Bad taste in the mouth
  - Sensitivity to light or sound
  - Mood changes or swings, agitation, combativeness, or other unusual behavior
  - Feeling anxious or depressed
  - Fatigue or drowsiness; a lack of energy or motivation

Headache, dizziness, confusion, and fatigue tend to start immediately after an injury, but resolve over time. Emotional symptoms, such as frustration and irritability tend to develop during recovery.

Traumatic Brain Injury in Children

Children might be unable to let others know that they feel different following a blow to the head. A child with a TBI may display the following signs or symptoms:

- Changes in eating or nursing habits
- Persistent crying, irritability, or crankiness; inability to be consoled
- Changes in ability to pay attention
- Lack of interest in a favorite toy or activity
- Changes in sleep patterns
- Seizures
- Sadness or depression
- Loss of a skill, such as toilet training
- Loss of balance or unsteady walking
- Vomiting

Effects on Consciousness

A TBI can cause problems with consciousness, awareness, alertness, and responsiveness. Generally, there are four abnormal states that can result from a severe TBI:

- **Minimally conscious state.** People with severely altered consciousness who still display some evidence of self-awareness or awareness of one's environment (such as following simple commands, yes/no responses).
- **Vegetative state.** A result of widespread damage to the brain, people in a vegetative state are unconscious and unaware of their surroundings. However, they can have periods of unresponsive alertness and may groan, move, or show reflex responses. If this state lasts longer than a few weeks, it is referred to as a "persistent vegetative state."

- **Coma.** A person in a coma is unconscious, unaware, and unable to respond to external stimuli, such as pain or light. Coma generally lasts a few days or weeks after which the person may regain consciousness, die, or move into a vegetative state.
- **Brain death.** The lack of measurable brain function and activity after an extended period of time is called "brain death" and may be confirmed by studies that show no blood flow to the brain.

WHAT ARE THE LEADING CAUSES OF TRAUMATIC BRAIN INJURY?

- **Falls.** According to data from the Centers for Disease Control and Prevention (CDC), falls are the most common cause of TBIs and occur most frequently among the youngest and oldest age groups. From 2006 to 2010 alone, falls caused more than half (55%) of TBIs among children 14 years of age and younger. Among Americans, 65 years of age and older, falls accounted for more than two-thirds (81%) of all reported TBIs.
- **Blunt trauma accidents.** Accidents that involve being struck by or against an object, particularly sports-related injuries, are a major cause of TBI. Anywhere from 1.6 million to 3.8 million sports- and recreation-related TBIs are estimated to occur in the United States annually.
- **Vehicle-related injuries.** Pedestrian-involved accidents, as well as accidents involving motor vehicles and bicycles, are the third most common cause of TBI. In young adults 15 to 24 years of age, motor vehicle accidents are the most likely cause of TBI.
- **Assaults/violence.** Assaults include abuse-related TBIs, such as head injuries that result from domestic violence or shaken baby syndrome, and gunshot wounds to the head. TBI-related deaths in children 4 years of age and younger are most likely the result of an assault.
- **Explosions/blasts.** TBIs caused by blast trauma from roadside bombs became a common injury to service

members in recent military conflicts. The majority of these TBIs were classified as mild head injuries.

- **Adults 65 years of age** and older are at greatest risk for being hospitalized and dying from a TBI, most likely from a fall. In every age group, serious TBI rates are higher for men than for women. Men are more likely to be hospitalized and are nearly three times more likely to die from a TBI than women.

HOW IS TRAUMATIC BRAIN INJURY DIAGNOSED?

All TBIs require immediate assessment by a professional who has experience evaluating head injuries. A neurological exam will judge motor and sensory skills and test hearing and speech, coordination and balance, mental status, and changes in mood or behavior, among other abilities. Screening tools for coaches and athletic trainers can identify the most concerning concussions for medical evaluation.

- **Initial assessments** may rely on standardized instruments, such as the Acute Concussion Evaluation (ACE) form from the Centers for Disease Control and Prevention or the Sport Concussion Assessment Tool 2, which provide a systematic way to assess a person who has suffered a mild TBI. Reviewers collect information about the characteristics of the injury, the presence of amnesia (loss of memory) and/or seizures, as well as the presence of physical, cognitive, emotional, and sleep-related symptoms. The ACE is also used to track symptom recovery over time. It also takes into account risk factors (including concussion, headache, and psychiatric history) that can impact how long it takes to recover from a TBI.
- **Diagnostic imaging**. When necessary, medical providers will use brain scans to evaluate the extent of the primary brain injuries and determine if surgery will be needed to help repair any damage to the brain. The need for imaging is based on a physical examination by a doctor and a person's symptoms.

- **Computed tomography (CT)** is the most commonly used imaging technology to assess people with suspected moderate to severe TBI. CT uses a series of x-rays (concentrated bursts of ionizing radiation) to create a two-dimensional image of organs, bones, and tissues and can show a skull fracture or any brain bruising, bleeding, or swelling.
- **Magnetic resonance imaging (MRI)** uses computer-generated radio waves and a powerful magnetic field to produce detailed images of body tissue. It may be used after the initial assessment and treatment as it is a more sensitive test and picks up subtle changes in the brain that the CT scan might have missed. Much of what is believed to occur to the brain following mild TBI happens at the cellular level. Significant advances have been made in the last decade to image milder TBI damage. For example, diffusion tensor imaging can image white matter tracts, more sensitive tests like fluid-attenuated inversion recovery can detect small areas of damage, and susceptibility-weighted imaging very sensitively identifies bleeding. Despite these improvements, currently available imaging technologies, blood tests, and other measures remain inadequate for detecting these changes in a way that can help diagnose mild concussive injuries.
- **Neuropsychological tests** to gauge brain functioning are often used in conjunction with imaging in people who have suffered mild TBI. Such tests involve performing specific cognitive tasks that help assess memory, concentration, information processing, executive functioning, reaction time, and problem solving. The Glasgow Coma Scale (GCS) is the most widely used tool for assessing the level of consciousness after TBI. The standardized 15-point test measures a person's ability to open her or his eyes and respond to spoken questions or physical prompts for movement. A

total score of 3 to 8 indicates a severe head injury; 9 to 12 indicates moderate injury; and 13 to 15 is classified as mild injury.

Many athletic organizations recommend establishing a baseline picture of an athlete's brain function at the beginning of each season, ideally before any head injuries have occurred. Baseline testing should begin as soon as a child begins a competitive sport. Brain function tests yield information about an individual's memory, attention, and ability to concentrate and solve problems. Brain function tests can be repeated at regular intervals (every 1 to 2 years) and also after a suspected concussion. The results may help healthcare providers identify any effects from an injury and allow them to make more informed decisions about whether a person is ready to return to their normal activities.

HOW IS TRAUMATIC BRAIN INJURY TREATED?

Many factors, including the size, severity, and location of the brain injury, influence how a TBI is treated and how quickly a person might recover. One of the critical elements to a person's prognosis is the severity of the injury. Although brain injury often occurs at the moment of head impact, much of the damage related to severe TBI develops from secondary injuries which happen days or weeks after the initial trauma. For this reason, people who receive immediate medical attention at a certified trauma center tend to have the best health outcomes.

Treating Mild Traumatic Brain Injury

Some people with mild TBI, such as concussion may not require treatment other than rest and over-the-counter (OTC) pain relievers. Treatment should focus on symptom relief and "brain rest." Monitoring by a healthcare practitioner is important to note any worsening of symptoms or new ones.

Children and teens who have a sports-related concussion should stop playing immediately and return to play only after being approved by a concussion injury specialist.

Preventing future concussions is critical. While most people recover fully from a first concussion within a few weeks, the rate of recovery from a second or third concussion is generally slower.

Even after symptoms resolve entirely, people should return to their daily activities gradually once they are given permission by a doctor. There is no clear timeline for a safe return to normal activities although there are guidelines, such as those from the American Academy of Neurology (AAN) and the American Medical Society for Sports Medicine (AMSSM) to help determine when athletes can return to practice or competition. Further research is needed to better understand the effects of mild TBI on the brain and to determine when it is safe to resume normal activities.

People with a mild TBI should make an appointment for a follow-up visit with their healthcare provider to confirm the progress of their recovery.

- Inquire about new or persistent symptoms and how to treat them.
- Pay attention to any new signs or symptoms even if they seem unrelated to the injury (for example, mood swings, unusual feelings of irritability).

These symptoms may be related even if they occurred several weeks after the injury.

Medications to treat some of the symptoms of TBI may include:

- OTC or prescribed pain medicines
- Anticonvulsant drugs to treat seizures
- Anticoagulants to prevent blood clots
- Diuretics to help reduce fluid buildup and reduce pressure in the brain
- Stimulants to increase alertness
- Antidepressants and antianxiety medications to treat depression and feelings of fear and nervousness

Treating Severe Traumatic Brain Injury

Immediate treatment for someone who has suffered a severe TBI focuses on preventing death; stabilizing the person's spinal cord, heart, lung, and other vital organ functions; ensuring proper oxygen delivery and breathing; controlling blood pressure; and preventing further brain damage. Emergency care staff also will monitor the flow of blood to the brain, brain temperature, pressure inside the skull, and the brain's oxygen supply.

Surgery may be needed for emergency medical care and to treat secondary damage, including:

- Relieving pressure inside the skull (inserting a special catheter through a hole drilled into the skull to drain fluids and relieve pressure)
- Removing debris or dead brain tissue (especially for penetrating TBI)
- Removing hematomas
- Repairing skull fractures

In-hospital strategies for managing people with severe TBI aim to prevent conditions including:

- Infection, particularly pneumonia
- Deep vein thrombosis (DVT) (blood clots that occur deep within a vein; risk increases during long periods of inactivity)

People with TBIs may need nutritional supplements to minimize the effects that vitamin, mineral, and other dietary deficiencies may cause over time. Some individuals may even require tube feeding to maintain the proper balance of nutrients.

Rehabilitation

After the acute care period of in-hospital treatment, people with severe TBI are often transferred to a rehabilitation center where a multidisciplinary team of healthcare providers help with recovery.

The rehabilitation team includes neurologists, nurses, psychologists, nutritionists, as well as physical, occupational, vocational, speech, and respiratory therapists.

Therapy is aimed at improving the person's ability to handle activities of daily living and to address cognitive, physical, occupational, and emotional difficulties. Treatment may be needed only short-term or throughout a person's life. Some therapy is provided through outpatient services.

Cognitive rehabilitation therapy (CRT) is a strategy aimed at helping individuals regain their normal brain function through an individualized training program. Using this strategy, people may also learn compensatory strategies for coping with persistent deficiencies involving memory, problem solving, and the thinking skills to get things done. CRT programs tend to be highly individualized and their success varies. A 2011 Institute of Medicine report concluded that cognitive rehabilitation interventions need to be developed and assessed more thoroughly.

Other Factors That Influence Recovery
GENES

Genetics may play a role in how quickly and completely a person recovers from a TBI. For example, researchers have found that apolipoprotein E ε4 (ApoE4)—a genetic variant associated with higher risks for Alzheimer disease (AD)—is associated with worse health outcomes following a TBI. Much work remains to be done to understand how genetic factors, as well as how specific types of head injuries, affect recovery. This research may lead to new treatment strategies and improved outcomes for people with TBI.

AGE

Studies suggest that age and the number of head injuries a person has suffered over her or his lifetime are two critical factors that impact recovery. For example, TBI-related brain swelling in children can be very different from the same condition in adults, even when the primary injuries are similar. Brain swelling in newborns, young infants, and teenagers often occurs much more quickly than it does in older individuals. Evidence from very limited CTE studies suggest that younger people (20 to 40 years of age) tend to have behavioral and mood changes associated with CTE, while those who are older (50+ years of age) have more cognitive difficulties.

Compared with younger adults with the same TBI severity, older adults are likely to have less complete recovery. Older people also have more medical issues and may often be taking multiple medications that may complicate treatment (e.g., blood-thinning agents when there is a risk of bleeding into the head). Further research is needed to determine if and how treatment strategies may need to be adjusted based on a person's age.

Researchers are continuing to look for additional factors that may help predict a person's course of recovery.

CAN TRAUMATIC BRAIN INJURY BE PREVENTED?

The best treatment for TBI is prevention. Unlike most neurological disorders, head injuries can be prevented. According to the CDC, doing the following can help prevent TBIs:

- Wear a seatbelt when you drive or ride in a motor vehicle.
- Wear the correct helmet and make sure it fits properly when riding a bicycle, skateboarding, and playing sports, such as hockey and football.
- Install window guards and stair safety gates at home for young children.
- Never drive under the influence of drugs or alcohol.
- Improve lighting and remove rugs, clutter, and other trip hazards in the hallway.
- Use nonslip mats and install grab bars next to the toilet and in the tub or shower for older adults.
- Install handrails on stairways.
- Improve balance and strength with a regular physical activity program.
- Ensure children's playgrounds are made of shock-absorbing material, such as hardwood mulch or sand.

Section 2.2 | **Classification of Traumatic Brain Injury**

This section includes text excerpted from "Traumatic Brain Injury in the United States: Epidemiology and Rehabilitation," Centers for Disease Control and Prevention (CDC), June 15, 2013. Reviewed May 2020.

The severity of traumatic brain injury (TBI) can be classified as mild, moderate, or severe on the basis of clinical presentation of a patient's neurologic signs and symptoms. The symptoms of TBI vary from one person to another, and although some symptoms might resolve completely, others, especially as a result of moderate and severe TBIs, can result in symptoms that persist, resulting in partial or permanent disability.

The assessment of TBI-related health effects is vital for the delivery of medical care, for discharge planning, inpatient treatment, and rehabilitation. Some health effects of TBI in children, such as deficits in organization and problem-solving might be delayed, and not surface until later. As a result, for both adults and children, TBI is being recognized more as a disease process, rather than a discrete event, because of the potential it presents for nonreversible and chronic health effects.

INJURY SEVERITY CLASSIFICATION OF TBI

Although several injury indicators exist for the classification of TBI, the Glasgow Coma Scale (GCS) is the most widely used. The GCS is a neurologic scale consisting of three components: eye-opening, verbal response, and motor response. The component scores are added to create an overall score to determine a patient's level of consciousness. The GCS was originally developed in 1974 to assess coma and other impaired levels of consciousness based on observed clinical signs and symptoms, but was later adopted to assess TBI severity. However, the GCS has some limitations. Factors not necessarily related to the injury might affect the GCS score and lead to misclassification of TBI severity. Some of these include factors that can independently alter consciousness, such as medical sedation, alcohol or drug intoxication, and organ system failure.

Traumatic brain injury severity can be misclassified when the GCS is used alone. Because of this, additional criteria are used in clinical practice and research.

These include duration of altered mental state or loss of consciousness and duration of posttraumatic amnesia. Imaging techniques, such as computed tomography (CT) scans, also can be used to identify structural damage that might contribute to the assessment of injury severity. In research studies, the Abbreviated Injury Scale (AIS) score for the head and neck region can be used to classify TBI. The AIS ranks injuries on a six-point scale based on mortality risk, with "1" indicating minor injury and "6" indicating a nonsurvivable injury. The relationship of these measures to classification of TBI severity as mild, moderate, or severe. However, as with the GCS, each of the severity criteria has limitations and might not be an accurate predictor of TBI severity and outcome when used alone.

Section 2.3 | Symptoms of Traumatic Brain Injury

This section includes text excerpted from "Symptoms of Traumatic Brain Injury (TBI)," Centers for Disease Control and Prevention (CDC), March 11, 2019.

WHAT ARE THE SYMPTOMS OF TRAUMATIC BRAIN INJURY?

Most people with a traumatic brain injury (TBI) recover well from symptoms experienced at the time of the injury. Most TBIs that occur each year are mild, commonly called "concussions," which is a mild TBI. But, for some people, symptoms can last for days, weeks, or longer. In general, recovery may be slower among older adults, young children, and teens. Those who have had a TBI in the past are also at risk of having another one. Some people may also find that it takes longer to recover if they have another TBI.

Symptoms Usually Fall into Four Categories

Some of these symptoms may appear right away. Others may not be noticed for days or months after the injury, or until the person resumes their everyday life. Sometimes, people do not recognize or admit that they are having problems. Others may not understand

Table 2.1. Four Categories of Symptoms

Thinking/ Remembering	Physical	Emotional/ Mood	Sleep
Difficulty thinking clearly	Headache Fuzzy or blurry vision	Irritability	Sleeping more than usual
Feeling slowed down	Nausea or vomiting(early on) Dizziness	Sadness	Sleep less than usual
Difficulty concentrating	Sensitivity to noise or light Balance problems	More emotional	Trouble falling asleep
Difficulty remembering new information	Feeling tired, having no energy	Nervousness or anxiety	

their problems and how the symptoms they are experiencing impact their daily activities.

The signs and symptoms of a concussion can be difficult to sort out. Early on, problems may be overlooked by the person with the concussion, family members, or doctors. People may look fine even though they are acting or feeling differently.

WHEN TO SEEK IMMEDIATE MEDICAL ATTENTION
Danger Signs in Adults

In rare cases, a dangerous blood clot that crowds the brain against the skull can develop. The people checking on you should take you to an emergency department (ED) right away if you have:

- Headache that gets worse and does not go away
- Weakness, numbness, or decreased coordination
- Repeated vomiting or nausea
- Slurred speech
- Look very drowsy or cannot wake up
- Have one pupil (the black part in the middle of the eye) larger than the other
- Have convulsions or seizures
- Cannot recognize people or places

- Are getting more and more confused, restless, or agitated
- Have unusual behavior
- Lose consciousness

Danger Signs in Children

Take your child to the emergency department (ED) right away if they received a bump, blow, or jolt to the head or body, and:

- Have any of the danger signs for adults listed above
- Will not stop crying and are inconsolable
- Will not nurse or eat

Section 2.4 | Potential Effects of Traumatic Brain Injury

This section contains text excerpted from the following sources: Text under the heading "What Are the Potential Effects of Traumatic Brain Injury?" is excerpted from "Potential Effects," Centers for Disease Control and Prevention (CDC), February 25, 2019; Text beginning with the heading "What Is Chronic Traumatic Encephalopathy? (CTE)" is excerpted from "Chronic Traumatic Encephalopathy (CTE)," Centers for Disease Control and Prevention (CDC), January 2019; Text under the heading "How Does Traumatic Brain Injury Affect the Brain?" is excerpted from "Traumatic Brain Injury—Hope Through Research," Centers for Disease Control and Prevention (CDC), September 2015. Reviewed May 2020.

WHAT ARE THE POTENTIAL EFFECTS OF TRAUMATIC BRAIN INJURY?

The severity of a traumatic brain injury (TBI) may range from "mild" (i.e., a brief change in mental status or consciousness) to "severe" (i.e., an extended period of unconsciousness or amnesia after the injury).

A TBI can cause a wide range of functional short- or long-term changes affecting:

- **Thinking** (i.e., memory and reasoning);
- **Sensation** (i.e., sight and balance);
- **Language** (i.e., communication, expression, and understanding); and
- **Emotion** (i.e., depression, anxiety, personality changes, aggression, acting out, and social inappropriateness).

29

A TBI can also cause epilepsy and increase the risk for conditions such as Alzheimer disease (AD), Parkinson disease (PD), and other brain disorders.

About 75 percent of TBIs that occur each year are concussions or other forms of mild TBI.

Repeated mild TBIs occurring over an extended period of time can result in cumulative neurological and cognitive deficits. Repeated mild TBIs occurring within a short period of time (i.e., hours, days, or weeks) can be catastrophic or fatal.

WHAT IS CHRONIC TRAUMATIC ENCEPHALOPATHY?

Chronic traumatic encephalopathy (CTE) is a brain disease that can only be diagnosed after death. It has been linked to specific changes in the brain that affect how the brain works. The research to date suggests that CTE is caused in part by repeated traumatic brain injuries, including concussions, and repeated hits to the head, called "subconcussive head impacts." However, understanding among researchers about the causes of CTE is currently limited. Researchers do not know the number and types of head impacts that increase the risk for CTE. It is possible that biological, environmental, or lifestyle factors could also contribute to the brain changes found in people with CTE diagnosed after death.

WHAT ARE SUBCONCUSSIVE HEAD IMPACTS?

Subconcussive head impacts are bumps, blows, or jolts to the head. Unlike concussions, which cause symptoms, subconcussive head impacts do not cause symptoms. A collision while playing sports is one way a person can get a subconcussive head impact.

HOW IS CHRONIC TRAUMATIC ENCEPHALOPATHY DIAGNOSED?

To diagnose CTE, doctors check the brain of a person after she or he dies. Doctors look for changes in the brain that happen in people with CTE. Through this process, doctors confirm whether the person had CTE or another disease, such as AD, or no disease at all. Given the limited understanding of CTE and its causes, doctors cannot diagnose CTE in a living person.

HOW COMMON IS CHRONIC TRAUMATIC ENCEPHALOPATHY?

Researchers do not know how many people in the United States have CTE. Most studies on CTE have focused on a small group of people who experienced head or brain injuries over many years. People in this group had their brains donated for research, and according to reports from family members, they often had problems with thinking, emotions, or behavior while they were alive.

Chronic traumatic encephalopathy has been diagnosed in people with and without a history of head or brain injuries. However, most people with a history of head or brain injuries do not develop CTE.

WHAT ARE THE SIGNS AND SYMPTOMS OF CHRONIC TRAUMATIC ENCEPHALOPATHY?

Researchers are not certain what symptoms are directly linked to CTE. Family members have reported noticing changes in thinking, feeling, behavior, and movement among people who are later diagnosed with CTE after death. Some people diagnosed with CTE first had problems with depression or anxiety. Some later developed memory and other thinking problems. Over time, some of these people had mood or personality changes. Family members of people who were later diagnosed with CTE have reported that their family member had problems that became serious enough to get in the way of normal daily activities (such as social or work-related activities).

The symptoms described by family members are similar to those of other health problems (e.g., AD, PD), so having these symptoms does not mean a person has CTE.

In addition, while there is increasing media attention on suicide among former professional athletes, the link between CTE and suicide is unclear.

If you or a family member or friend have any questions or concerns, it is important to talk to a doctor. Treatments are available to help with many of these symptoms.

HOW DOES TRAUMATIC BRAIN INJURY AFFECT THE BRAIN?

Traumatic brain injury-related damage can be confined to one area of the brain, known as a "focal injury," or it can occur over a more widespread area, known as a "diffuse injury." The type of injury is another determinant of the effect on the brain. Some injuries are considered primary, meaning the damage is immediate. Other consequences of TBI can be secondary, meaning they can occur gradually over the course of hours, days, or weeks. These secondary brain injuries are the result of reactive processes that occur after the initial head trauma.

There are a variety of immediate effects on the brain, including various types of bleeding and tearing forces that injure nerve fibers and cause inflammation, metabolic changes, and brain swelling.

- Diffuse axonal injury (DAI) is one of the most common types of brain injuries. DAI refers to widespread damage to the brain's white matter. White matter is composed of bundles of axons (projections of nerve cells that carry electrical impulses). Like the wires in a computer, axons connect various areas of the brain to one another. DAI is the result of shearing forces, which stretch or tear these axon bundles. This damage commonly occurs in auto accidents, falls, or sports injuries. It usually results from rotational forces (twisting) or sudden deceleration. It can result in a disruption of neural circuits and a breakdown of overall communication among nerve cells, or neurons, in the brain. It also leads to the release of brain chemicals that can cause further damage. These injuries can cause temporary or permanent damage to the brain, and recovery can be prolonged.

- Concussion—a type of mild TBI that may be considered a temporary injury to the brain but could take minutes to several months to heal. Concussion can be caused by a number of things, including a bump, blow, or jolt to the head, sports injury or fall, motor vehicle accident, weapons blast, or a rapid acceleration or deceleration of the brain within the skull (such as the person having been violently shaken). The individual either suddenly loses consciousness or has a sudden altered state of consciousness or awareness, and is often called "dazed" or said to have her/his "bell rung." A second concussion closely following the first one causes further damage to the brain—the so-called "second hit" phenomenon—and can lead to permanent damage or even death in some instances.

- Hematomas—a pooling of blood in the tissues outside of the blood vessels. Hematomas can develop when major blood vessels in the head become damaged, causing severe bleeding in and around the brain. Different types of hematomas form depending on where the blood collects relative to the meninges. The meninges are the protective membranes surrounding the brain, which consist of three layers: dura mater (outermost), arachnoid mater (middle), and pia mater (innermost).

  - **Epidural hematomas** involve bleeding into the area between the skull and the dura mater. These can occur with a delay of minutes to hours after a skull fracture damages an artery under the skull, and are particularly dangerous.
  - **Subdural hematomas** involve bleeding between the dura and the arachnoid mater, and, like epidural hematomas, exert pressure on the outside of the brain. Their effects vary depending on their size. They are very common in the elderly after a fall.
  - **Subarachnoid hemorrhage** is bleeding that occurs between the arachnoid mater and the pia mater and their effects vary depending on their size.
  - **Bleeding into the brain** itself is called an "intracerebral hematoma" and damages the surrounding tissue.

- Contusions—a bruising or swelling of the brain that occurs when very small blood vessels bleed into brain tissue. Contusions can occur directly under the impact site (i.e., a coup injury) or, more often, on the complete opposite side of the brain from the impact (i.e., a contrecoup injury). They can appear after a delay of hours to a day. Coup/Contrecoup lesions—contusions or subdural hematomas that occur at the site of head impact as well as directly opposite the coup lesion. Generally they occur when the head abruptly decelerates, which causes the brain to bounce back and forth within the skull (such as in a high-speed car crash). This type of injury also occurs in shaken baby syndrome, a severe head injury that results when an infant or toddler is shaken forcibly enough to cause the brain to bounce back and forth against the skull.
- Skull fractures—breaks or cracks in one or more of the bones that form the skull. They are a result of blunt force trauma and can cause damage to the underlying areas of the skull such as the membranes, blood vessels, and brain. One main benefit of helmets is to prevent skull fracture.

The first 24 hours after mild TBI are particularly important because subdural hematoma, epidural hematoma, contusion, or excessive brain swelling (edema) are possible and can cause further damage. For this reason doctors suggest watching a person for changes for 24 hours after a concussion.

- Hemorrhagic progression of a contusion (HPC) contributes to secondary injuries. HPCs occur when an initial contusion from the primary injury continues to bleed and expand over time. This creates a new or larger lesion—an area of tissue that has been damaged through injury or disease. This increased exposure to blood, which is toxic to brain cells, leads to swelling and further brain cell loss.

- Secondary damage may also be caused by a breakdown in the blood-brain barrier. The blood-brain barrier preserves the separation between the brain fluid and the very small capillaries that bring the brain nutrients and oxygen through the blood. Once disrupted, blood, plasma proteins, and other foreign substances leak into the space between neurons in the brain and trigger a chain reaction that causes the brain to swell. It also causes multiple biological systems to go into overdrive, including inflammatory responses which can be harmful to the body if they continue for an extended period of time. It also permits the release of neurotransmitters, chemicals used by brain cells to communicate, which can damage or kill nerve cells when depleted or overexpressed.
- Poor blood flow to the brain can also cause secondary damage. When the brain sustains a powerful blow, swelling occurs just as it would in other parts of the body. Because the skull cannot expand, the brain tissue swells and the pressure inside the skull rises; this is known as "intracranial pressure" (ICP). When the intracranial pressure becomes too high it prevents blood from flowing to the brain, which deprives it of the oxygen it needs to function. This can permanently damage brain function.

Chapter 3 | **Concussion and Brain Injury**

WHAT IS A CONCUSSION?

A concussion is a type of traumatic brain injury—or TBI—caused by a bump, blow, or jolt to the head or by a hit to the body that causes the head and brain to move rapidly back and forth. This sudden movement can cause the brain to bounce around or twist in the skull, creating chemical changes in the brain and sometimes stretching and damaging brain cells.

Concussions Are Serious

Medical providers may describe a concussion as a "mild" brain injury because concussions are usually not life-threatening. Even so, the effects of a concussion can be serious.

CONCUSSION SIGNS AND SYMPTOMS

Children and teens who show or report one or more of the signs and symptoms listed below, or simply say they just "don't feel right" after a bump, blow, or jolt to the head or body may have a concussion or more serious brain injury.

Concussion Signs Observed

- Cannot recall events prior to or after a hit or fall
- Appears dazed or stunned

This chapter includes text excerpted from "Brain Injury Basics" Centers for Disease Control and Prevention (CDC), March 5, 2019.

- Forgets an instruction, is confused about an assignment or position, or is unsure of the game, score, or opponent
- Moves clumsily
- Answers questions slowly
- Loses consciousness (even briefly)
- Shows mood, behavior, or personality changes

Concussion Symptoms Reported
- Headache or "pressure" in head
- Nausea or vomiting
- Balance problems or dizziness, or double or blurry vision
- Bothered by light or noise
- Feeling sluggish, hazy, foggy, or groggy
- Confusion, or concentration or memory problems
- Just not "feeling right," or "feeling down"

Signs and symptoms generally show up soon after the injury. However, you may not know how serious the injury is at first and some symptoms may not show up for hours or days. For example, in the first few minutes, your child or teen might be a little confused or a bit dazed, but an hour later your child might not be able to remember how she or he got hurt.

You should continue to check for signs of concussion right after the injury and a few days after the injury. If your child or teen's concussion signs or symptoms get worse, you should take her or him to the emergency department right away.

CONCUSSION DANGER SIGNS
In rare cases, a dangerous collection of blood (hematoma) may form on the brain after a bump, blow, or jolt to the head or body that may squeeze the brain against the skull. Call 911 right away, or take your child or teen to the emergency department if she or he has one or more of the following danger signs after a bump, blow, or jolt to the head or body:

Dangerous Signs and Symptoms of a Concussion
- One pupil larger than the other.

- Drowsiness or inability to wake up.
- A headache that gets worse and does not go away.
- Slurred speech, weakness, numbness, or decreased coordination.
- Repeated vomiting or nausea, convulsions or seizures (shaking or twitching).
- Unusual behavior, increased confusion, restlessness, or agitation.
- Loss of consciousness (passed out/knocked out). Even a brief loss of consciousness should be taken seriously.

Dangerous Signs and Symptoms of a Concussion for Toddlers and Infants

- Any of the signs and symptoms listed in the danger signs and symptoms of a concussion list.
- Will not stop crying and cannot be consoled.
- Will not nurse or eat.

Chapter 4 | Severe Traumatic Brain Injury

Each year, traumatic brain injury (TBI) causes a substantial number of deaths and leads to life-long disability for many Americans. In fact, TBIs contribute to about 30 percent of all injury deaths in the United States. In 2014, there were:

- Approximately 2.5 million TBI-related emergency department visits,
- Approximately more than 288,000 hospitalizations, and
- Nearly 57,000 deaths related to TBI.

The effects of a TBI can vary significantly, depending on the severity. Individuals with a mild TBI generally experience short-term symptoms and feel better within a couple of weeks, whereas individuals with a moderate or severe TBI may have long-term or life-long effects from the injury.

A severe TBI not only impacts the life of an individual and their family, but it also has a large societal and economic toll. The life-time economic cost of TBI, including direct and indirect medical costs, was estimated to be approximately $76.5 billion (in 2010 dollars). Additionally, the cost of fatal TBIs and TBIs requiring hospitalization, many of which are severe, account for approximately 90 percent of total TBI medical costs. Falls are one of the leading causes of TBI-related emergency department (ED) visits, hospitalizations, and deaths, and recent data shows that over half of fall-related TBIs were among the youngest (0 to 4 years of age) and oldest age groups (≥75 years of age).

This chapter includes text excerpted from "Severe TBI," Centers for Disease Control and Prevention (CDC), April 2, 2019.

POTENTIAL EFFECTS OF SEVERE TRAUMATIC BRAIN INJURY

The long-term effects of a TBI have been described as being similar to the effects of chronic disease. Individuals who experience mild TBI are more likely to recover from their initial injury symptoms, although some individuals experience longer-term effects. Individuals who experience more severe TBI are more likely to have lasting effects from the injury.

A TBI may lead to a wide range of short- or long-term issues affecting:

- **Cognitive function** (attention and memory)
- **Motor function** (extremity weakness, impaired coordination, and balance)
- **Sensation** (hearing, vision, impaired perception, and touch)
- **Behavior** (emotional regulation, depression, anxiety, aggression, impairments in behavioral control, personality changes)

A severe TBI may lead to death, or result in an extended period of unconsciousness (coma) or amnesia. Individuals may experience significant changes in thinking and behavior. Moderate-to-severe TBI may also result in a reduced lifespan.

The consequences of severe TBI can affect all aspects of an individual's life, including relationships with family and friends, the ability to progress at school or work, doing household tasks, driving, or participating in other daily activities.

TRAUMATIC BRAIN INJURY IN THE MILITARY

Blasts are a leading cause of TBI for active duty military personnel in war zones. The Centers for Disease Control and Prevention (CDC) estimates of TBI do not include injuries seen in the U.S. Department of Defense (DOD) or the U.S. Veterans Health Administration Hospitals (VHA).

RESEARCH AND PREVENTION

While there is no one size fits all solution, there are interventions and programs that can be effective to help limit the impact of severe

TBI. These measures include prevention, early management, and treatment.

The CDC's research and programs work to reduce TBI and its consequences by developing and evaluating clinical guidelines, conducting surveillance, implementing primary prevention and education strategies, and developing evidence-based interventions to save lives and reduce the long-term effects of TBI.

Developing and Evaluating Clinical Guidelines

The CDC researchers conducted a study to assess the effectiveness of adopting the Brain Trauma Foundation (BTF) in hospital guidelines for the treatment of adults with severe traumatic brain injury (TBI). This research indicated widespread adoption of these guidelines could result in:

- A 50 percent decrease in deaths
- A savings of approximately $288 million in medical and rehabilitation costs
- A savings of approximately $3.8 billion to society

Implementing Prevention and Education Strategies

The CDC has multiple education and awareness efforts to help improve primary prevention of TBI, as well as those that promote early identification and appropriate care.

- **Fall prevention strategies.** Healthcare providers can reduce their older patients' chances of falling by implementing strategies from the Stopping Elderly Accidents, Deaths, and Injuries, or STEADI, initiative.
- **Motor vehicle safety strategies.**
  - Child passenger safety depends on increased car seat and booster seat use. Child restraint laws, enhanced enforcement, incentives, and education programs are among the strategies recommended.
  - Strategies to increase seat belt use include primary seat belt laws, increased penalties, and short-term, high visibility enforcement.

- **The MyMobility Plan** provides older adults with information, guidance, and tips on how to stay safe, mobile, and independent as they age.
- **Strategies to prevent or reduce drunk driving** include drunk driving laws, sobriety checkpoints, and ignition interlocks.

Conducting Surveillance

Surveillance data are critical to help inform prevention strategies, identify modifiable risk and protective factors, and identify trends to let us know whether the problem is getting better or worse (and whether prevention efforts are working).

Chapter 5 | High-Risk Groups for Brain Injury

Chapter Contents

Section 5.1 | **Pediatric Traumatic Brain Injury**

This section includes text excerpted from "The Management of Traumatic Brain Injury in Children: Opportunities for Action," Centers for Disease Control and Prevention (CDC), March 25, 2020.

INCIDENCE

Traumatic brain injury (TBI) in children represents a significant public-health burden in the United States.

A TBI disrupts the normal function of the brain, and can be caused by a bump, blow, or jolt to the head, or a penetrating head injury.

In 2013, there were approximately 640,000 TBI-related emergency department (ED) visits, 18,000 TBI-related hospitalizations, and 1,500 TBI-related deaths among children 14 years of age and younger. The leading cause of TBI-related ED visits, hospitalizations, and deaths for those 0 to 14 years of age were unintentional falls and being struck by or against an object, whereas for those 15 to 24 years of age the leading causes were motor vehicle crashes and falls. Sports and recreation-related TBIs are a leading cause of TBI-related ED visits among children and teens with an estimated 325,000 which occurred in 2012.

Children with TBI can present to a number of clinical locations: the ED, urgent care clinics, primary care, concussion/sports medicine clinics, or other specialty clinics. In addition, some do not seek or receive medical care. Research examining the point of entry in a large healthcare network found that among pediatric patients with mild TBI (mTBI), 82 percent initially visited primary care, 5 percent visited specialty care, and 12 percent visited an ED. This incidence estimates of pediatric TBI based solely on ED visit data are significant undercounts, likely missing those with mTBIs seen at lower levels of care, in addition to those with mTBIs who do not seek care at all. Because of these gaps in TBI surveillance, researchers have found it difficult to accurately estimate the true incidence of pediatric TBI, a critical factor in understanding the public-health burden it represents.

Rates of TBI-related deaths and TBI-related hospitalizations among children have decreased in recent years (i.e., from 2007 to 2013). However, TBI-related ED visits among children have significantly increased during the same time period. More specifically, ED visits as a result of TBIs experienced during sports and recreational activities have increased. The increase in ED visits may not be a true increase in incidence, but rather a response to increased public concern about concussion, resulting in a higher likelihood of seeking care, improved training of clinicians in concussion diagnosis, and the passage of legislation in all 50 states requiring healthcare provider clearance prior to a child returning to play.

INJURY SEVERITY

Traumatic brain injury severity is typically separated into categories of mild, moderate, and severe based on a patient's initial clinical presentation, and is measured by behavioral indicators, primarily the Glasgow Coma Scale (GSC), and the pediatric coma scale (PCS). As defined by the GSC, a score of 13 to 15 is labeled an mTBI, a score of 8 to 12 is labeled a moderate TBI, and a score less than 8 is labeled a severe TBI. Complicated mTBI is a designation given when a child has a mild GSC rating (13 to 15) with neuro-imaging findings (e.g., skull fracture, intracranial bleeding) on the day of injury. The presence of a visible abnormality on imaging suggests greater neuropathology in the child's brain at the time of injury, although the long-term effects of such documented changes on children's brain structure and outcomes are mixed. The concept of mTBI is thus viewed as a continuum when imaging findings are included in the severity ratings.

Most TBIs are mild, and are commonly called "concussions." From this point forward, we will refer to concussions as mTBI). Mild TBI accounts for 70 to 90 percent of TBI-related ED visits. In a study of children seeking emergency medical care from hospitals for TBI (N=2940), 84.5 percent had mTBI, 13.2 percent had moderate TBI, and 2.3 percent had severe TBI. Moderate-to-severe TBI occurs at a lower rate than mTBI in children, but is associated with worse outcomes. In addition, African American, Hispanic,

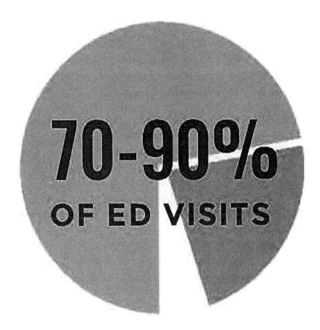

Figure 5.1. Total Mild Traumatic Brain Injury (mTBI) Accounts

and Native American children are more likely than white children to experience more severe TBI, and have higher mortality rates.

MECHANISM OF INJURY

The cause, or mechanism of TBI, is an important consideration in understanding its epidemiology because the mechanisms of injury suggest the types of events that need to be prevented. The leading mechanisms of TBI vary by age, but falls, motor-vehicle crashes, and sports and recreation-related injuries are the primary mechanisms of injury in children.

Falls are the leading cause of TBI-related ED visits in the youngest children (0 to 4 years of age), accounting for more than 70 percent of TBI-related ED visits in this age group in 2013. Injuries caused by falls (35.1%) and being struck by, or against an object account for the majority of TBI-related ED visits among youth 5 to 14 years of age. For people in the 15 to 24 years age group,

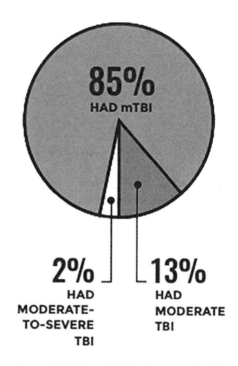

85%
HAD mTBI

2% ⌐ ⌐**13%**
HAD ... HAD
MODERATE- ... MODERATE
TO-SEVERE ... TBI
TBI

Figure 5.2. Children's Seeking Emergency Medical Care in Hospital for Traumatic Brain Injury (TBI)

the proportions of TBI-related ED visits resulting from assaults, falls, and motor vehicle events are nearly equal. African American, Hispanic, and Native American children are more likely than white children to experience a TBI caused by violence or to be struck by a motor vehicle while walking or bicycling.

In 2012, approximately 430,000 ED visits resulted from sports and recreation-related mTBI. Nearly 70 percent of those ED visits (3,25,000) were among those 0 to 19 years of age. From 2001 to 2012 the rate of sports and recreation-related ED visits increased significantly among males, particularly among those 10 to 14 years of age (139.9% increase) and those 15 to 19 years of age (119.3% increase). Among males, the largest number of ED visits for sports and recreation-related mTBI occurred as a result of injuries while bicycling, or playing football or basketball. A similar increase was found for females, particularly among those 15 to 19 years of age

(211.5% increase) and those 10 to 14 years of age (145.2% increase). Among females 0 to 19 years of age, the largest number of ED visits for sports and recreation-related mTBIs occurred as a result of injuries while bicycling, engaging in playground activities, or horseback riding. In addition to sports-related injuries, the rate of ED visits for playground-related TBIs significantly increased from 2005 to 2013.

During 2001 to 2013, an annual average of 21,201 children 14 years of age and younger were seen in the ED for playground-related TBIs. The highest rates of playground-related TBIs were found among males and children 5 to 9 years of age.

Abusive head trauma (AHT) in children is a mechanism of injury most frequently experienced by young children, and it generally results in moderate or severe injury. Annual estimates of AHT ED visits and hospital admissions from 2001 to 2006 were 3,227 nationally; nearly two-thirds of those visits resulted in hospital admission, a reflection of the typical severity of AHT.

THE EFFECTS OF TRAUMATIC BRAIN INJURY IN CHILDREN

Adults with moderate-to-severe TBI who receive inpatient rehabilitation typically experience significant changes in critical aspects of their daily life. These include higher rates of unemployment, disability, and even a reduced life expectancy. However, children, who are in the midst of significant brain development, differ greatly from adolescents and adults in brain biomechanics, pathophysiology, and neurodevelopment. Injuries of any severity to the developing brain can negatively impact children's behavior and cognitive skills as they grow, placing them at risk for significant changes to their developmental trajectory across multiple domains. An additional consideration is that children typically recover well in relation to the outward physical manifestations of the injury (e.g., physical skills), but may have sustained damage to their brain, affecting thinking and behavior that is often not visible. The "invisible" nature of a TBI may lead to unmet care needs and difficulties with meeting societal expectations, resulting in misattribution of an individual's behavior, and discrimination.

To date, little research has examined long-term adult outcomes following a childhood TBI. In particular, it is unclear how changes in brain development and skill attainment caused by a TBI in childhood impacts achievement in adult metrics such as educational attainment, employment, and adult health. The burden of TBI in children can be explained by examining disability, participation limitations, economic impact, and disparities in healthcare.

Section 5.2 | Head Injury due to Fall in Elderly

This section includes text excerpted from "Important Facts about Falls," Centers for Disease Control and Prevention (CDC), February 10, 2017.

Each year, millions of older people—those 65 years of age and older—fall. In fact, more than one in four older people falls each year, but less than half tell their doctor. Falling once doubles your chances of falling again.

FALLS ARE SERIOUS AND COSTLY

- One in five falls causes a serious injury, such as broken bones or a head injury.
- Each year, 3 million older people are treated in emergency departments for fall injuries.
- Over 800,000 patients a year are hospitalized because of a fall injury, most often because of a head injury or hip fracture.
- Each year at least 300,000 older people are hospitalized for hip fractures.
- More than 95 percent of hip fractures are caused by falling, usually by falling sideways.
- Falls are the most common cause of traumatic brain injury (TBI).
- In 2015, the total medical costs for falls totaled more than $50 billion. Medicare and Medicaid shouldered 75 percent of these costs.

WHAT CAN HAPPEN AFTER A FALL?

Many falls do not cause injuries. But, one in five falls does cause a serious injury, such as a broken bone or a head injury. These injuries can make it hard for a person to get around, do everyday activities, or live on their own.

- Falls can cause broken bones such as wrist, arm, ankle, and hip fractures
- Falls can cause head injuries. These can be very serious, especially if the person is taking certain medicines (like blood thinners). An older person who falls and hits their head should see their doctor right away to make sure they do not have a brain injury.
- Many people who fall, even if they are not injured, become afraid of falling. This fear may cause a person to cut down on their everyday activities. When a person is less active, they become weaker and this increases their chances of falling.

WHAT CONDITIONS MAKE YOU MORE LIKELY TO FALL?

Research has identified many conditions that contribute to falling. These are called "risk factors." Many risk factors can be changed or modified to help prevent falls. They include:

- Lower body weakness
- Vitamin D deficiency (that is, not enough vitamin D in your system)
- Difficulties with walking and balance
- Use of medicines such as tranquilizers, sedatives, or antidepressants. Even some over-the-counter (OTC) medicines can affect balance and how steady you are on your feet.
- Vision problems
- Foot pain or poor footwear
- Home hazards or dangers such as:
  - Broken or uneven steps
  - Throw rugs or clutter that can be tripped over

Most falls are caused by a combination of risk factors. The more risk factors a person has, the greater their chances of falling.

Healthcare providers can help cut down a person's risk by reducing the fall risk factors listed above.

What You Can Do to Prevent Falls

Falls can be prevented. These are some simple things you can do to keep yourself from falling.

TALK TO YOUR DOCTOR

- Ask your doctor or healthcare provider to evaluate your risk for falling and talk with them about specific things you can do.
- Ask your doctor or pharmacist to review your medicines to see if any of them might make you dizzy or sleepy. This should include prescription medicines and OTC medicines.
- Ask your doctor or healthcare provider about taking vitamin D supplements.

DO STRENGTH AND BALANCE EXERCISES

Do exercises that make your legs stronger and improve your balance. Tai Chi is a good example of this kind of exercise.

HAVE YOUR EYES CHECKED

Have your eyes checked by an eye doctor at least once a year, and be sure to update your eyeglasses if needed.

If you have bifocal or progressive lenses, you may want to get a pair of glasses with only your distance prescription for outdoor activities, such as walking. Sometimes these types of lenses can make things seem closer or farther away than they really are.

MAKE YOUR HOME SAFER

- Get rid of things you could trip over.
- Add grab bars inside and outside your tub or shower and next to the toilet.

- Put railings on both sides of stairs.
- Make sure your home has lots of light by adding more or brighter light bulbs.

Section 5.3 | Domestic Abuse and Traumatic Brain Injury

"Domestic Abuse and Traumatic Brain Injury," © 2016 Omnigraphics. Reviewed May 2020.

Traumatic brain injury (TBI) is a type of damage to the brain that results from an external physical force being applied to the head. TBI may occur when the head strikes a stationary object, such as the ground or a wall, or when the head is struck by a hard object, such as a baseball bat. TBI can also result from forceful shaking of the head, which causes the brain to move around within the skull, or from penetration of the skull by a foreign object, such as a bullet or a knife. Brain injury may also occur from the deprivation of oxygen through choking or near-drowning.

Although media attention has raised awareness of the risk of TBI among athletes and military veterans, little consideration has been given to the prevalence of TBI among women who are survivors of domestic violence. Yet research has shown that 90 percent of all injuries from domestic violence occur to the face, head, or neck. One study found that 30 percent of women who sought emergency medical treatment for domestic violence injuries had lost consciousness at least once, and 67 percent showed symptoms of TBI. Another study found that 75 percent of the battered women in three domestic violence shelters reported receiving a brain injury from an intimate partner, while 50 percent had sustained multiple brain injuries.

Many of the common acts of physical aggression that are used by perpetrators of domestic violence can cause brain injuries, including beating someone on the head with fists or other objects, pushing someone downstairs or into a solid object, shaking someone strenuously, choking or holding someone underwater, and shooting or stabbing someone in the face or head. Victims of domestic violence may not realize that they have sustained a brain injury, especially if they do not seek or receive medical treatment. But, a history of TBI leads to a substantially greater risk of sustaining further brain injuries, and repeated brain injuries are known to have a cumulative effect.

EFFECTS OF TRAUMATIC BRAIN INJURY

Traumatic brain injury affects people differently, so the symptoms may vary depending on the individual. There are some initial symptoms that are fairly common, however, including a brief loss of consciousness, dizziness, headaches, loss of short-term memory, slower processing of information, fatigue, and sensitivity to light and sound. With repeated injuries or lack of medical treatment, people with TBI may experience increased levels of physical, cognitive, and functional disabilities. Some of the most common problems include:

- Weakness, clumsiness, and motor control difficulties
- Communication difficulties, including slurring of speech and problems with word-finding
- Issues involving balance, vision, and hearing
- Difficulty concentrating or paying attention, along with increased distractibility
- Issues with problem-solving and task completion
- Difficulty with long-term goal setting, prioritizing, planning, and organization
- Increased tension, anxiety, and irritability
- Impulsiveness and lapses in judgment
- Increased risk of depression and substance abuse

Survivors of domestic violence may experience a wide range of challenges related to TBI. Slower reaction time and inattentiveness, for instance, may increase the risk that physical abuse will result in further brain injuries. Abusive partners may also try to use the symptoms of a brain injury as tools to manipulate and control their victims. For instance, they may take advantage of short-term memory loss to make victims doubt their memories and perceptions of past abuse.

Survivors with TBI may also find it more difficult to assess situations, make plans for their own safety, leave an abusive partner, and live independently or in a domestic violence shelter. They may also have trouble accessing support services, remembering appointments, and navigating the criminal justice system. Testifying in child custody or criminal court proceedings requires survivors to remember details of abuse and communicate them clearly and sequentially. Yet these abilities may be compromised in individuals with TBI, which may reduce their credibility in court and negatively affect their outcomes. Domestic violence survivors with TBI may also experience problems caring for children or maintaining employment.

SUPPORTING SURVIVORS WITH TRAUMATIC BRAIN INJURY

Advocates and service providers for survivors of domestic violence must be aware of the high risk of TBI among their clients. Shelters and counseling facilities should put screening procedures in place to identify people with TBI, train staff to address their special needs and challenges, and implement organizational policies to better support them. Some additional tips for helping domestic violence survivors with TBI include:

- Treat people as individuals. Strive to understand and accommodate their unique challenges and strengths, provide positive and respectful feedback, and empower them to make necessary changes in their lives.
- Be aware that an abuse survivor may have TBI even in the absence of a formal diagnosis. If TBI has been diagnosed, however, do not assume that the individual has cognitive or functional disabilities.
- Recognize that behavioral concerns and noncompliance with shelter rules may be linked to an underlying TBI. Provide accommodations as needed— such as a planner to help a person with memory deficits remember communal responsibilities—to enable abuse survivors to adapt to the shelter environment.
- Keep in mind that recovery from a brain injury takes time and does not necessarily happen in a linear or

57

sequential manner. As a result, people's needs may change frequently.

- Adapt safety planning to make it more appropriate for people living with TBI. Many safety planning discussions require domestic violence survivors to envision hypothetical circumstances or remember long lists of actions to be executed in a crisis. But, these discussions can be challenging for people with TBI who struggle with abstract thought or memory problems. To make the discussions more productive, experts recommend minimizing outside distractions, holding shorter meetings more frequently, focusing on a single topic at each meeting, making action items simple and concrete, and concluding by summarizing the information and checking for understanding.
- Educate others about TBI and its intersection with domestic violence.

References

1. "The Intersection of Brain Injury and Domestic Violence," New York State Coalition Against Domestic Violence, n.d.
2. "Traumatic Brain Injury and Domestic Violence Facts," Alabama Department of Rehabilitation Services, 2012.

Section 5.4 | Traumatic Brain Injury, Drug Addiction, and the Developing Teen Brain

This section includes text excerpted from "Traumatic Brain Injury, Drug Addiction, and the Developing Teen Brain," National Institute on Drug Abuse (NIDA) for Teens, March 19, 2015. Reviewed May 2020.

Nowadays, when there are news reports about traumatic brain injury (TBI), it is almost always related to football. And while one of the effects of TBI is an increased risk of using drugs and alcohol (especially for teens), this chapter is not really about that.

THE DEVELOPING TEEN BRAIN: WHY IT IS AT RISK

We have talked a lot about why drug use is so dangerous in your teen years—that it raises your risk for being addicted. The teen brain is still developing—growing—and this makes it more flexible, more impressionable. So what you do now has a big impact on who you become as an adult. Like molding clay before it hardens, or programming a computer, you are wiring your brain.

It turns out that the developing brain is also at high risk for concussions, which doctors call "mild TBIs" (mTBIs). Concussions can cause people to feel confused and depressed, to have a hard time remembering events around the time of the injury, to get headaches and seizures, and possibly to lose consciousness (pass out).

TRAUMATIC BRAIN INJURY AND THE DEVELOPING TEEN BRAIN

Compared with adults, children and teens have large heads in relation to their necks (like a bobblehead) and their brains' nerve fibers can be torn apart more easily. So children and teens have a greater chance of getting a concussion. Many young people recover rapidly, but the younger a person is, the longer it can take to recover. Sometimes, young people have more serious effects from TBIs compared to adults.

It is not just age that makes a difference; research from the past few years has shown that girls are at a greater risk for concussions than boys, and girls' brains need more time to recover than previously thought.

Every concussion is different. When two heads slam together (inside helmets or not) or a ball hits your head, it can force your brain out of its protective fluid, slamming it against your skull and shaking it. It can disrupt how your brain works—for a few seconds, minutes, hours, days, weeks, months, years, or forever.

The nature of the injury, where it happens in the brain, the individual characteristics of the person's brain, and the environment all play a role in how bad the damage is. And people who get a concussion and go back to playing too soon are at risk of getting additional concussions more easily, and possibly having much more severe outcomes. In rare cases, this can even cause death.

TRAUMATIC BRAIN INJURY AND DRUGS: PROTECT YOURSELF

Traumatic brain injury poses higher risks for the teen brain because it is still being formed. This is also one of the reasons that using drugs as a teen increases the chances for addiction—the brain is simply more vulnerable while it is developing.

March is Brain Injury Awareness Month. Take precautions to protect your brain. Seat belts and helmets can save your life. But, if you do get a concussion, listen to your doctor and force yourself to rest for the full time prescribed, even when you feel ready to get back to the sport you love. And remember, there is no helmet for drugs. So protect your brain inside and out.

Section 5.5 | Traumatic Brain Injury in Prisoners

This section includes text excerpted from "Traumatic Brain Injury in Prisons and Jails," Centers for Disease Control and Prevention (CDC), 2011. Reviewed May 2020.

Many people in prisons and jails are living with traumatic brain injury (TBI)-related problems that complicate their management and treatment while they are incarcerated. Because most prisoners will be released, these problems will also pose challenges when they return to the community. The Centers for Disease Control and Prevention (CDC) recognizes TBI in prisons and jails as an important public-health problem.

WHAT IS KNOWN ABOUT TRAUMATIC BRAIN INJURY AND RELATED PROBLEMS IN PRISONS AND JAILS?
General

- More than two million people currently reside in U.S. prisons and jails.
- According to jail and prison studies, 25 to 87 percent of inmates report having experienced a head injury or TBI as compared to 8.5 percent in a general population reporting a history of TBI.

- Prisoners who have had head injuries may also experience mental-health problems such as severe depression and anxiety, substance use disorders, difficulty controlling anger, or suicidal thoughts and/or attempts.

Women
- Although women are outnumbered by men in U.S. prisons and jails, their numbers more than doubled from 1990 to 2000. As of June 2005, more than 200,000 women were incarcerated. Women now represent 7 percent of the total U.S. prison population and 12 percent of the total U.S. jail population.
- Women inmates who are convicted of violent crime are more likely to have sustained a precrime TBI and/or some other form of physical abuse.
- Women with substance use disorders have an increased risk for TBI compared with other women in the general U.S. population.
- Preliminary results from one study suggest that TBI among women in prison is very common.

Substance Abuse, Violence, and Homelessness
- Studies of prisoners' self-reported health indicate that those with one or more head injuries have significantly higher levels of alcohol and/or drug use during the year preceding their current incarceration.
- The U.S. Department of Justice (DOJ) has reported that 52 percent of female offenders and 41 percent of male offenders are under the influence of drugs, alcohol, or both at the time of their arrest and that 64 percent of male arrestees tested positive for at least one of five illicit drugs (cocaine, opioids, marijuana, methamphetamines, or phencyclidine (PCP).
- Among male prisoners, a history of TBI is strongly associated with the perpetration of domestic and other kinds of violence.

- Children and teenagers who have been convicted of a crime are more likely to have had a precrime TBI and/or some other kind of physical abuse.
- Homelessness has been found to be related to both head injury and prior imprisonment.

HOW DO TRAUMATIC BRAIN INJURY-RELATED PROBLEMS AFFECT PRISONERS WITH TRAUMATIC BRAIN INJURY AND OTHERS DURING THEIR INCARCERATION?

A TBI may cause many different problems:

- Attention deficits may make it difficult for the prisoner with TBI to focus on a required task or respond to directions given by a correctional officer. Either situation may be misinterpreted, thus leading to an impression of deliberate defiance on the part of the prisoner.
- Memory deficits can make it difficult to understand or remember rules or directions, which can lead to disciplinary actions by jail or prison staff.
- Irritability or anger might be difficult to control and can lead to an incident with another prisoner or correctional officer and to further injury for the person and others.
- Slowed verbal and physical responses may be interpreted by correctional officers as uncooperative behavior.
- Uninhibited or impulsive behavior, including problems controlling anger and unacceptable sexual behavior, may provoke other prisoners or result in disciplinary action by jail or prison staff.

WHAT IS NEEDED TO ADDRESS THE PROBLEM OF TRAUMATIC BRAIN INJURY IN JAILS AND PRISONS?

A recent report from the Commission on Safety and Abuse in America's Prisons recommends increased health screenings, evaluations, and treatment for inmates.

In addition, TBI experts and some prison officials have suggested:

- Routine screening of jail and prison inmates to identify a history of TBI.
- Screening inmates with TBI for possible alcohol and/ or substance abuse and appropriate treatment for these co-occurring conditions.
- Additional evaluations to identify specific TBI-related problems and determine how they should be managed. Special attention should be given to impulsive behavior, including violence, sexual behavior, and suicide risk if the inmate is depressed.

WHAT IS NEEDED TO ADDRESS TRAUMATIC BRAIN INJURY RELATED PROBLEMS AFTER RELEASE FROM JAILS AND PRISONS?

Lack of treatment and rehabilitation for people with mental health and substance abuse problems while incarcerated increases the probability that they will again abuse alcohol and/or drugs when released. Persistent substance problems can lead to homelessness, return the drug to illegal activities, rearrests, and increase the risk of death after release. As a result, criminal justice professionals and TBI experts have suggested the following:

- Community re-entry staff should be trained to identify a history of TBI and have access to appropriate consultation with other professionals with expertise in TBI.
- Transition services for released people returning to communities should accommodate the problems resulting from a TBI.
- Released people with mental health and/or substance abuse problems should receive case management services and assistance with placement into community treatment programs.

The CDC supports new research to develop better methods for identifying inmates with a history of TBI and related problems and for determining how many of them are living with such injury.

Chapter 6 | **TBI: Facts and Statistics**

Traumatic brain injury (TBI) is a major cause of death and disability in the United States. From 2006 to 2014, the number of TBI-related emergency department visits, hospitalizations, and deaths (EDHDs) increased by 53 percent. In 2014, an average of 155 people in the United States died each day from injuries that include a TBI. Those who survive a TBI can face effects that last a few days, or the rest of their lives. Effects of TBI can include impairments related to thinking or memory, movement, sensation (e.g., vision or hearing), or emotional functioning (e.g., personality changes, depression). These issues not only affect individuals but also can have lasting effects on families and communities.

HOW BIG IS THE PROBLEM?
- In 2014, about 2.87 million TBI-related emergency department visits, hospitalizations, and deaths occurred in the United States, including over 837,000 of these health events among children.
  - TBI contributed to the deaths of 56,800 people, including 2,529 deaths among children.
  - TBI was diagnosed in approximately 288,000 hospitalizations, including over 23,000 among children. These consisted of TBI alone or TBI in combination with other injuries.

This chapter contains text excerpted from the following sources: Text in this chapter begins with excerpts from "TBI: Get the Facts," Centers for Disease Control and Prevention (CDC), March 11, 2019; Text beginning with the heading "Traumatic Brain Injury-Related Emergency Department Visits, Hospitalizations, and Deaths" is excerpted from "TBI Data and Statistics," Centers for Disease Control and Prevention (CDC), March 29, 2019.

- In 2014, an estimated 812,000 children (17 years of age or younger) were treated in the United States in the EDs for concussion or TBI, alone or in combination with other injuries.
- Over the span of eight years (2006–2014), while age-adjusted rates of TBI-related ED visits increased by 54 percent, hospitalization rates decreased by 8 percent and death rates decreased by 6 percent.

CAUSES OF TRAUMTIC BRAIN INJURY

- In 2014, falls were the leading cause of TBI. Falls accounted for almost half (48%) of all TBI-related emergency department visits. Falls disproportionately affect children and older adults:
  - Almost half (49%) of TBI-related ED visits among children 0 to 17 years were caused by falls.
  - Four in five (81%) TBI-related ED visits in older adults aged 65 years and older were caused by falls
- Being struck by or against an object was the second leading cause of TBI-related ED visits, accounting for about 17% of all TBI-related ED visits in the United States in 2014.
- Over 1 in 4 (28%) TBI-related ED visits in children less than 17 years of age or less were caused by being struck by or against an object.
- Falls and motor vehicle crashes were the first and second leading causes of all TBI-related hospitalizations (52% and 20%, respectively).
- Intentional self-harm was the first leading cause of TBI-related deaths (33%) in 2014.

RISK FACTORS OF TRAUMATIC BRAIN INJURY

Among TBI-related deaths in 2014:
- Rates were highest for persons 75 years of age and older.
- The leading cause of TBI-related death varied by age:
  - Falls were the leading cause of death for persons 65 years of age or older.

- Intentional self-harm was the leading cause of death for persons 45-64 years of age.
- Motor vehicle crashes were the leading cause of death for persons 15-24, 25-34, and older adults ≥75 years of age.
- Homicide was the leading cause of death for children 0-4 years of age.
- Among TBI-related ED visits and hospitalizations in 2014:
- Hospitalization rates were highest among persons 75 years of age and older.
- Rates of ED visits were highest for persons 75 years of age and older and children 0-4 years of age.
- The leading cause of TBI-related ED visits varied by age:
  - Falls were the leading cause of ED visits among young children 0 to 4 years of age and older adults 65 years and older.
  - Being struck by or against an object was highest among those 5 to 14 years of age.
- The leading cause of TBI-related hospitalizations varied by age:
  - Falls were the leading cause of hospitalizations among children 0 to 17 years and adults 55 years of age and older.
  - Motor vehicle crashes were the leading cause of hospitalizations for adolescents and adults aged 15 to 44 years of age.

TRAUMATIC BRAIN INJURY-RELATED EMERGENCY DEPARTMENT VISITS, HOSPITALIZATIONS, AND DEATHS

In 2014, there were approximately 2.87 million TBI-Emergency Department Visits, Hospitalizations, and Deaths (EDHDs) in the United States, including over 837,000 occurring among children. This includes:

- Approximately 2.53 million TBI-related ED visits, including over 812,00 occurring among children.

Table 6.1. EDHD-Data Table

	2006	2007	2008	2009	2010	2011	2012	2013	2014
Emergency Department Visits, Hospitalizations, and Deaths total	1,884,195	1,925,173	2,019,166	2,377,868	2,521,966	2,653,617	2,735,909	2,797,754	2,877,757
Emergency department visits	1,551,107	1,603,124	1,698,326	2,047,886	2,143,133	2,332,299	2,390,167	2,460,278	2,532,537
Hospitalizations	278,655	267,350	267,015	277,315	325,996	267,480	290,360	281,555	288,420
Deaths	54,433	54,699	53,825	52,667	52,837	53,837	55,382	55,921	56,800

Healthcare Cost and Utilization Project's (HCUP) Nationwide Emergency Department Sample for emergency department visits; HCUP's Nationwide Inpatient Sample for hospitalizations; the Centers for Disease Control and Prevention (CDC), National Vital Statistics System for deaths

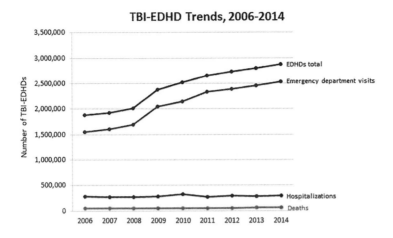

Figure 6.1. Rates of Traumatic Brain Injury-Emergency Department Visits, Hospitalizations, and Deaths Trends, 2006 to 2014.

- Approximately 288,000 TBI-related hospitalizations, including over 23,000 occurring among children.
- 56,800 TBI-related deaths, including 2,529 occurring among children.

Traumatic Brain Injury-Emergency Department Visits, Hospitalizations, and Deaths Trends

- The number of total TBI-EDHDs increased by 53 percent from 2006 (N approximately 1.88 million) to 2014 (N approximately 2.88 million).

TRAUMATIC BRAIN INJURY-RELATED EMERGENCY DEPARTMENT VISITS

- In 2014, there were approximately 2.5 million TBI-related Emergency Department (ED) visits in the United States, including over 812,000 among children.
- Unintentional falls, being unintentionally struck by or against an object, and motor vehicle crashes were the most common mechanisms of injury contributing to a TBI

Rates of TBI-ED Visits, By Mechanism of Injury, 2006-2014

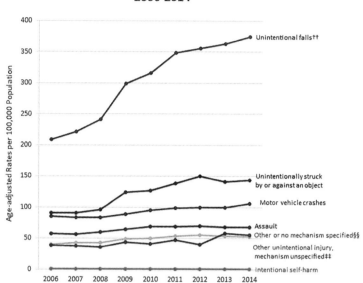

Figure 6.2. Rates of Traumatic Brain Injury-Related Emergency Department Visits by Mechanism of Injury 2006 to 2014.

diagnosis in the ED. These three principal mechanisms of injury accounted for 47.9 percent, 17.1 percent, and 13.2 percent, respectively, of all TBI-related ED visits.

- Rates of TBI-related ED visits per 100,000 population were highest among adults 75 years of age and older (1,682.0), young children 0 to 4 years of age (1,618.6), and individuals 15 to 24 years of age (1,010.1).

Trends in Age-Adjusted Rates of Traumatic Brain Injury-Related Emergency Department Visits

- Age-adjusted rates of TBI-related ED visits increased 54 percent from 521.6 per 100,000 population in 2006 to 801.9 in 2014. An increase in age-adjusted rates occurred among nearly all of the major unintentional and intentional principal mechanism categories, including:

Table 6.2. Age-Adjusted Rates of Traumatic Brain Injury-Related Emergency Department Visits, Mechanism of Injury 2006 to 2014-Data Table

	2006	2007	2008	2009	2010	2011	2012	2013	2014
Motor vehicle crashes	85.3	83.8	83.9	88.7	95.3	98.7	99.9	99.6	106
Unintentional falls††	208.8	221.7	240.9	298.8	316.3	348.7	355.9	362.9	374.9
Unintentionally struck by or against an object	90.8	90.6	95.8	123.9	127	138.8	149.8	141	143.9
Other unintentional injuries, mechanism unspecified‡‡	40.4	42.7	43.1	49.5	50.5	53.4	55.4	54.1	53.2
Intentional self-harm	0.5	0.4	0.5	0.6	0.6	0.7	0.7	0.7	0.8
Assault	57.6	56.8	60.3	64.6	68.7	68.9	69.9	68	67.8
Other or no mechanism specified§§	38.2	37.7	35.3	44.2	41.1	47.1	40.4	58.3	55.3
Total	521.6	533.8	559.8	670.2	699.5	756.3	771.9	784.6	801.9

Source: Healthcare Cost and Utilization Project's (HCUP) Nationwide Emergency Department Sample. Age-adjusted to the 2000 U.S. standard population. ††Includes falls of undetermined intent to maintain consistency with past data releases. ‡‡E-codes specify that the injury was unintentional but do not specify the actual mechanism of injury. §§Includes TBIs in which the intent was not determined as well as those due to legal intervention or war. Includes TBIs in which no mechanism was specified in the record. Does not include falls of undetermined intent.

- A 24 percent increase for TBI-related ED visits as a result of motor vehicle crashes (from 85.3 to 106);
- An 80 percent increase for TBI-related ED visits as a result of falls (from 208.8 to 374.9);

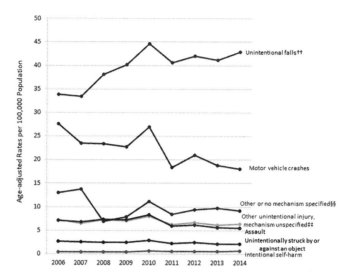

Figure 6.3. Rates of Traumatic Brain Injury-Related Hospitalizations by Mechanism of Injury 2006 to 2014.

- A 58 percent increase for TBI-related ED visits as a result of being struck by or against an object (from 90.8 to 143.9);
- A 60 percent increase for TBI-related ed visits as a result of intentional self-harm (from 0.5 to 0.8); and
- An 18 percent increase for TBIs as a result of assault (from 57.6 to 67.8).

TRAUMATIC BRAIN INJURY-RELATED HOSPITALIZATIONS

- In 2014, there were approximately 288,000 TBI-related hospitalizations in the United States, including over 23,000 among children.
- Unintentional falls and motor vehicle crashes were the most common mechanisms of injury contributing to a TBI diagnosis in which the patient was hospitalized. These two principal mechanisms of injury accounted for 52.3

TBI: Facts and Statistics

Table 6.3. Age-Adjusted Rates of Traumatic Brain Injury-Related Hospitalizations, Mechanism of Injury 2006 to 2014-Data Table

	2006	2007	2008	2009	2010	2011	2012	2013	2014
Motor vehicle crashes	27.6	23.5	23.4	22.7	27	18.4	21	18.8	18.1
Unintentional falls††	33.9	33.5	38.1	40.2	44.6	40.6	42	41.2	42.9
Unintentionally struck by or against an object	2.7	2.6	2.5	2.5	2.9	2.3	2.5	2.2	2.2
Other unintentional injury, mechanism unspecified‡‡	7.3	6.5	7.2	7	8	6.3	6.7	6.2	6.4
Intentional self-harm	0.4	0.4	0.4	0.4	0.6	0.5	0.5	0.5	0.6
Assault	7.1	6.8	7.4	7.2	8.3	6	6.2	5.6	5.5
Other or no mechanism specified§§	13	13.8	6.9	7.9	11.2	8.4	9.4	9.7	9.2
Total	92.2	87.2	85.8	87.9	102.5	82.5	88.4	84.2	84.9

Source: Healthcare Cost and Utilization Project's (HCUP) Nationwide Inpatient Sample.
Age-adjusted to the 2000 U.S. standard population. ††Includes falls of undetermined intent to maintain consistency with past data releases. ‡‡E-codes specify that the injury was unintentional but do not specify the actual mechanism of injury. §§Includes TBIs in which the intent was not determined as well as those due to legal intervention or war. Includes TBIs in which no mechanism was specified in the record. Does not include falls of undetermined intent.

percent and 20.4 percent, respectively, of all TBI-related hospitalizations.
- Rates of TBI-related hospitalizations per 100,000 population were highest among adults 75 years of age and older (470.6), those 65 to 74 years of age (145.5), and individuals 55 to 64 years of age (89.5).

Rates of TBI-Deaths, By Mechanism of Injury, 2006-2014

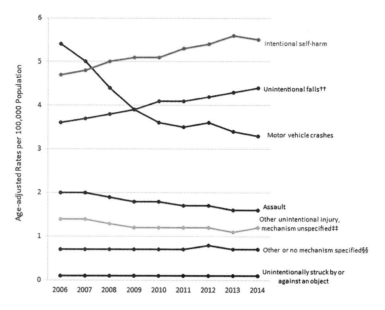

Figure 6.4. Traumatic Brain Injury-Related Deaths by Mechanism of Injury 2006 to 2014.

Trends in Age-Adjusted Rates of Traumatic Brain Injury-Related Hospitalizations

- From 2006 to 2014, age-adjusted rates of TBI-related hospitalizations decreased by nearly 8 percent (from 92.2 per 100,000 population to 84.9).
- This decrease coincides with a 34 percent decrease in the age-adjusted rate of TBI-related hospitalizations attributable to motor vehicle crashes (27.6 in 2006 to 18.1 in 2014).
- Despite the overall decrease in TBI-related hospitalization rates, there were increases in the age-adjusted rates of TBI-related hospitalizations attributable to falls (33.9 in 2006 to 42.9 in 2014) and intentional self-harm (0.4 in 2006 to 0.6 in 2014).

Table 6.4. Traumatic Brain Injury-Related Deaths by Mechanism of Injury 2006 to 2014-Data Table

	2006	2007	2008	2009	2010	2011	2012	2013	2014
Motor vehicle crashes	5.4	5	4.4	3.9	3.6	3.5	3.6	3.4	3.3
Unintentional falls††	3.6	3.7	3.8	3.9	4.1	4.1	4.2	4.3	4.4
Unintentionally struck by or against an object	0.1	0.1	0.1	0.1	0.1	0.1	0.1	0.1	0.1
Other unintentional injury, mechanism unspecified‡‡	1.4	1.4	1.3	1.2	1.2	1.2	1.2	1.1	1.2
Intentional self-harm	4.7	4.8	5	5.1	5.1	5.3	5.4	5.6	5.5
Assault	2	2	1.9	1.8	1.8	1.7	1.7	1.6	1.6
Other or no mechanism specified§§	0.7	0.7	0.7	0.7	0.7	0.7	0.8	0.7	0.7
Total	17.9	17.8	17.2	16.6	17.2	16.5	16.8	16.8	16.8

(Source: The Centers for Disease Control and Prevention (CDC) National Vital Statistics System. Age-adjusted to the 2000 U.S. standard population.)
Includes falls of undetermined intent to maintain consistency with past data releases. ‡‡E-codes specify that the injury was unintentional but do not specify the actual mechanism of injury. §§Includes TBIs in which the intent was not determined as well as those due to legal intervention or war. Includes TBIs in which no mechanism was specified in the record. Does not include falls of undetermined intent.

TRENDS IN AGE-ADJUSTED RATES OF TRAUMATIC BRAIN INJURY-RELATED DEATHS

- From 2006 to 2014, age-adjusted rates of TBI-related deaths decreased by 6 percent (from 17.9 per 100,000 population to 16.8).

- This decrease coincides with a large decrease in the age-adjusted rate of TBI-related deaths attributable to motor vehicle crashes (5.4 in 2006 to 3.3 in 2014).
- From 2006 to 2014, age-adjusted rates of TBI-related deaths attributable to falls and intentional self-harm increased (from 3.6 to 4.4 and from 4.7 to 5.5, respectively).

Part 2 | Diagnosis and Treatment of Traumatic Brain Injury

Chapter 7 | Traumatic Brain Injury: Seek Immediate Medical Attention

WHEN TO SEEK IMMEDIATE MEDICAL ATTENTION
Danger Signs in Adults

In rare cases, a dangerous blood clot that crowds the brain against the skull can develop. The people checking on you should take you to an emergency department (ED) right away if you have:

- Headache that gets worse and does not go away
- Weakness, numbness, or decreased coordination
- Repeated vomiting or nausea
- Slurred speech
- Look very drowsy or cannot wake up
- Have one pupil (the black part in the middle of the eye) larger than the other
- Have convulsions or seizures
- Cannot recognize people or places
- Are getting more and more confused, restless, or agitated
- Have unusual behavior
- Lose consciousness

This chapter contains text excerpted from the following sources: Text under the heading "When to Seek Immediate Medical Attention" is excerpted from "Symptoms of Traumatic Brain Injury (TBI)," Centers for Disease Control and Prevention (CDC), March 11, 2019; Text under the heading "What to Expect When You See a Healthcare Professional" is excerpted from "Response," Centers for Disease Control and Prevention (CDC), February 25, 2019.

Danger Signs in Children

Take your child to the emergency department (ED) right away if they received a bump, blow, or jolt to the head or body, and:

- Have any of the danger signs for adults listed above
- Will not stop crying and are inconsolable
- Will not nurse or eat

WHAT TO EXPECT WHEN YOU SEE A HEALTHCARE PROFESSIONAL

While most people are seen in an ED or medical office, some people must stay in the hospital overnight. Your healthcare professional may do a scan of your brain (such as a computed tomography (CT) scan) or other tests. Additional tests might be necessary such as tests of your learning, memory concentration, and problem-solving. These tests are called "neuropsychological" or "neurocognitive" tests and can help your healthcare professional identify the effects of a concussion. Even if the concussion does not show up on these tests, you may still have a concussion.

Your healthcare professional will send you home with important instructions to follow. Be sure to follow all of your healthcare professional's instructions carefully.

If you are taking medications—prescription, over-the-counter (OTC) medicines, or "natural remedies"—or if you drink alcohol or take illicit drugs, tell your healthcare professional. Also, tell your healthcare professional if you are taking blood thinners (anticoagulant drugs), such as Coumadin and aspirin, because they can increase the chance of complications.

Chapter 8 | **Diagnosis of Traumatic Brain Injury**

AN OVERVIEW OF TBI DIAGNOSIS[1]

While it can be hard to formally diagnose traumatic brain injury (TBI), the Centers for Disease Control and Prevention (CDC), the American College of Rehabilitation Medicine (ACRM), and some others have published guidelines for diagnosing TBI.

A medical exam is the first step in diagnosing potential head injury. Assessment usually includes a neurological exam. This exam includes an evaluation of thinking, motor function (movement), sensory function, coordination, and reflexes.

HOW DO HEALTHCARE PROVIDERS DIAGNOSE TRAUMATIC BRAIN INJURY?[2]
Glasgow Coma Scale

The Glasgow Coma Scale (GCS) measures a person's functioning in three areas:

- **Ability to speak,** such as whether the person speaks normally, speaks in a way that does not make sense, or does not speak at all
- **Ability to open eyes,** including whether the person opens her or his eyes only when asked
- **Ability to move,** ranging from moving one's arms easily to not moving even in response to painful stimulation

This chapter includes text excerpted from documents published by two public domain sources. Text under headings marked 1 are excerpted from "Traumatic Brain Injury: What to Know about Symptoms, Diagnosis, and Treatment," U.S. Food and Drug Administration (FDA), March 20, 2019; Text under headings marked 2 are excerpted from "How Do Health Care Providers Diagnose Traumatic Brain Injury (TBI)?" *Eunice Kennedy Shriver* National Institute of Child Health and Human Development (NICHD), December 1, 2016. Reviewed May 2020.

A healthcare provider rates a person's responses in these categories and calculates a total score. A score of 13 and higher indicates a mild TBI, 9 through 12 indicates a moderate TBI, and 8 or below indicates severe TBI. However, there may be no correlation between initial GCS score and the person's short- or long-term recovery or abilities.

Measurements for Level of Traumatic Brain Injury

Healthcare providers sometimes rank the person's level of consciousness, memory loss, and GCS score.

A TBI is considered mild if:
- The person was not unconscious or was unconscious for less than 30 minutes.
- Memory loss lasted less than 24 hours.
- The GCS was 13 to 15.

The National Institute of Child Health and Human Development (NICHD)-supported research has found, however, that diagnosis of mild TBI (concussion), in practice, uses inconsistent criteria and relies heavily on patients' self-reported symptoms.

A TBI is considered moderate if:
- The person was unconscious for more than 30 minutes and up to 24 hours.
- Memory loss lasted anywhere from 24 hours to 7 days.
- The GCS was 9 to 12.

A TBI is considered severe if:
- The person was unconscious for more than 24 hours.
- Memory loss lasted more than 7 days.
- The GCS was 8 or lower.

Speech and Language Tests
- A speech-language pathologist completes a formal evaluation of speech and language skills, including an oral motor evaluation of the strength and coordination of the muscles that control speech, understanding, and

use of grammar and vocabulary, as well as reading and writing.
- Social communication skills are evaluated with formal tests and role-playing scenarios.
- If a patient has problems with swallowing, the speech-language pathologist will make recommendations regarding management and treatment to ensure that the individual is able to swallow safely and receive adequate nutrition.

Cognition and Neuropsychological Tests
- **Cognition** describes the processes of thinking, reasoning, problem-solving, information processing, and memory.
  - Most patients with severe TBI suffer from cognitive disabilities, including the loss of many higher-level mental skills.
- **Neuropsychological** assessments are often used to obtain information about cognitive capabilities.
  - These tests are specialized task-oriented evaluations of human brain-behavior relationships, evaluating higher cognitive functioning as well as basic sensory-motor processes.
  - Testing by a neuropsychologist can assess the individual's cognitive, language, behavioral, motor, and executive functions and provide information regarding the need for rehabilitative services.
  - For this assessment, a neuropsychologist reviews the case history and hospital records of the patient, and interviews the patient and her or his family.
  - The neuropsychologist acquires information about the "person" the individual was before the injury, based on aspects such as school performance, habits, and lifestyle, in order to detail which abilities remain unchanged as well as areas of the brain that are adversely affected by the injury and how the injury is expected to impact the individual's life.

Imaging Tests

Healthcare providers may also use tests that take images of a person's brain. These include, but are not limited to:

- **Computerized tomography (CT).** A CT (or computerized axial tomography (CAT)) scan takes x-rays from many angles to create a complete picture. It can quickly show bleeding in the brain, bruised brain tissue, and other damage.
- **Magnetic resonance imaging (MRI).** MRI uses magnets and radio waves to produce more detailed images than CT scans. An MRI likely would not be used as part of an initial TBI assessment because it takes too long to complete. It may be used in follow-up examinations, though.
- **Intracranial pressure (ICP) monitoring.** Sometimes, swelling of the brain from a TBI can increase pressure inside the skull. The pressure can cause additional damage to the brain. A healthcare provider may insert a probe through the skull to monitor this swelling. In some cases, a shunt or drain is placed into the skull to relieve ICP.

TESTS FOR ASSESSING TRAUMATIC BRAIN INJURY IN MILITARY SETTINGS[2]

A severe trauma may be obvious in a military situation, but a milder TBI may not be as easy to identify. The U.S. Department of Defense (DOD) and Department of Veterans Affairs (VA) have, therefore, established procedures to assess quickly whether the person suffered:

- A loss of consciousness
- Memory problems
- Neurologic symptoms, such as confusion or poor coordination

This assessment, combined with other measures, helps determine the type of care necessary, including evacuation for a higher level of treatment.

SAFETY NOTE[1]

During recent monitoring of the medical device market, the U.S. Food and Drug Administration (FDA) became aware of some firms marketing medical devices for the assessment, diagnosis, or management of a head injury (including concussion) without proper FDA clearance or approval.

Medical devices that are not FDA-approved or FDA-cleared may not correctly diagnose a concussion. And incorrect diagnosis may lead to:

- A wrong decision to let a person return to play or other activities with a serious head injury
- A missed diagnosis of a more serious head injury
- The lack of proper treatment for a head injury

The FDA issued a Safety Communication in April 2019 to caution about the serious risks of using unapproved or uncleared medical devices for the diagnosis, treatment or management of a concussion.

The bottom line: if you have a head injury, seek medical attention right away. The FDA has not approved any devices that can assess or diagnose a concussion without an evaluation by a healthcare provider.

MORE FDA ACTIONS AND RESEARCH ON TBI[1]

The FDA continues to work with the research and clinical community to develop better-designed clinical studies so new medical products can be developed. And it continues to review and evaluate medical devices for safety and effectiveness.

More sensitive and objective ways to diagnose and detect mild TBI are needed. And timely diagnosis is important to prevent repetitive injury and to help develop new therapies. That is because repetitive injury carries the risk of "second impact syndrome." If people who have not recovered from a head injury have a second head injury, this can result in more significant injury to the brain and more neurological deficits. And, in some cases, repetitive injury can be fatal.

The FDA continues to research diagnostic tests for mild TBI. They are studying TBI biomarkers (measurable, biological indicators of a particular state or condition), such as brain imaging, biofluid (specific proteins in blood), and physical indicators such as eye tracking and electroencephalogram (EEG), which tracks and records brain wave patterns. They are also investigating using other portable imaging devices to detect mild TBI, including diffuse correlation spectroscopy—a device that can monitor blood flows in the brain from the scalp.

Plus, the FDA's scientists are doing research with patients at Walter Reed National Military Medical Center in Bethesda, Maryland. They are recruiting more adult patients—including those with and without TBI—for continued research.

Chapter 9 | **Treatment of Traumatic Brain Injury**

A variety of treatments can help promote recovery from the physical, emotional, and cognitive problems traumatic brain injury (TBI) may cause. The types and extent of treatments depend on the severity of the injury and its specific location in the brain.

TREATMENT FOR MILD TRAUMATIC BRAIN INJURY

Mild TBI, sometimes called "concussion," may not require specific treatment other than rest. However, it is very important to follow a healthcare provider's instructions for complete rest and gradual return to normal activities after a mild TBI. If a person resumes normal activities and starts experiencing TBI symptoms, the healing and recovery process may take much longer than if she or he had followed the health provider's instructions. Certain activities, such as working on a computer and concentrating hard, can tire the brain even though they are not physically demanding. The person with the concussion might need to reduce these kinds of activities or might need to rest between periods of such activities to let the brain rest. In addition, alcohol and other drugs can slow recovery and increase the chances of reinjury.

Children and teens who may have sustained a concussion during sports should stop playing immediately. They should not return to play until a healthcare provider who is experienced in evaluating concussion confirms they are ready. Reinjury during recovery can slow healing and increase the chances of long-term problems. On

This chapter includes text excerpted from "What Are the Treatments for TBI?" *Eunice Kennedy Shriver* National Institute of Child Health and Human Development (NICHD), December 1, 2016. Reviewed May 2020.

rare occasions in which a person gets another concussion before healing from the first one, permanent brain damage and even death may result.

EMERGENCY TREATMENT FOR TRAUMATIC BRAIN INJURY

In most cases, emergency care focuses on stabilizing the patient and promoting survival. This care may include ensuring adequate oxygen flow to the brain, controlling blood pressure, and preventing further injury to the head or neck. Once the patient is stable, other types of care for TBI and its effects can begin.

Surgery may be needed as part of emergency care to reduce additional damage to the brain tissues. Surgery may include:

- **Removing clotted blood**. Bleeding in the brain or between the brain and skull can lead to large areas of clotted blood, sometimes called "hematomas," that put pressure on the brain and damage brain tissues.
- **Repairing skull fractures**. Setting severe skull fractures or removing pieces of skull or other debris from the brain can help start the healing process of the skull and surrounding tissues.
- **Relieving pressure in the skull**. Making a hole in the skull or adding a shunt or drain can relieve pressure inside the skull and allow excess fluid to drain.

MEDICATIONS TO TREAT TRAUMATIC BRAIN INJURY

Medications may be used to treat symptoms of TBI and to lower some of the risks associated with it. These medications may include, but are not limited to:

- **Antianxiety medication** to lessen feelings of nervousness and fear
- **Anticoagulants** to prevent blood clots
- **Anticonvulsants** to prevent seizures
- **Antidepressants** to treat symptoms of depression and mood instability
- **Muscle** relaxants to reduce muscle spasms
- **Stimulants** to increase alertness and attention

Researchers continue to explore medications that may aid recovery from TBI. For example, an National Institute of Child Health and Human Development (NICHD) study investigated the effectiveness of citicoline, a drug meant to help protect neurological functioning. The study found, however, that patients with TBI who took citicoline did not have any greater improvement in function than those who took a placebo.

REHABILITATION THERAPIES FOR TRAUMATIC BRAIN INJURY

Therapies can help someone with TBI relearn skills, such as walking or cooking, or develop strategies for self-care, such as making lists of the steps involved in getting dressed. Rehabilitation can include several different kinds of therapy for physical, emotional, and cognitive difficulties. Depending on the injury, these treatments may be needed only briefly after the injury, occasionally throughout a person's life, or on an ongoing basis.

Types of Therapies for Traumatic Brain Injury

Most people with a moderate to severe brain injury will need some type of rehabilitation therapy to address physical, emotional, and cognitive issues from the TBI. Therapies will likely include relearning old skills or learning new ways to make up for lost skills. A treatment program should be designed to meet each person's specific needs and to strengthen her or his ability to function at home and in the community.

Therapy usually begins in the hospital and can continue in a number of possible settings, including in a skilled nursing facility, at home, in a school, and in an outpatient program at a clinic. Therapy can be brief or long-term, depending on the type of injury, and it may need to change over time. Rehabilitation generally involves a number of healthcare specialists, the person's family, and a person who manages the team. When devising a long-term treatment plan, patients, their families, and their providers should be aware that moderate and severe TBI impairs patients' ability to make sound medical decisions even a month after injury.

Types of rehabilitation therapy may include:
- **Physical therapy.** This treatment works to build physical strength, coordination, and flexibility.
- **Occupational therapy.** An occupational therapist helps a person learn or relearn how to perform daily tasks such as getting dressed, cooking, and bathing.
- **Speech therapy.** This therapy works on the ability to form words and other communication skills as well as how to use special communication devices if necessary. Speech therapy can also include evaluation and treatment of swallowing disorders (dysphagia).
- **Psychological counseling.** A counselor can help a person learn coping skills, work on relationships, and improve general emotional well-being.
- **Vocational counseling.** This type of rehabilitation focuses on a person's ability to return to work, find appropriate opportunities, and deal with workplace challenges.
- **Cognitive therapy.** This includes activities designed to improve memory, attention, perception, learning, planning, and judgment. For many people with TBI, cognitive therapy is among the most common types of rehabilitation.

Chapter 10 | **Surgical Options for Traumatic Brain Injury**

A blow to the head or a head injury that disrupts the normal function of the brain is known as a "traumatic brain injury" (TBI). It is usually caused when an object pierces the skull and enters the brain tissue. Depending on the extent of damage to the brain, the symptoms of a TBI can be mild, moderate, or severe. Major cases of TBI may result in longer periods of unconsciousness, coma, or even death. TBI is a major risk factor for injury-related mortality globally. Every year, 1.7 million cases of TBI occur in the United States, and around 5.3 million people live with a disability caused by TBI.

The surgical treatment of TBI is challenging, and the two major types of surgery performed to treat TBI are explained below.

DECOMPRESSIVE CRANIECTOMY

A brain surgery that involves removing a portion of the skull is known as a "decompressive craniectomy." The pressure in the brain can build up within the skull when the brain swells after an injury, causing more damage; this being the reason to perform a decompressive craniectomy.

The Procedure

The hair over the damaged portion of the scalp is shaved. The patient is then made unconscious by inducing general anesthesia.

"Surgical Options for Traumatic Brain Injury," © 2020 Omnigraphics. Reviewed May 2020.

The neurosurgeon cuts the skin and underlying tissues, revealing the skull. The neurosurgeon then removes a portion of the skull (usually the area that covers the injury) that causes pressure to the brain. As the skull is a hard bone, a drill and bone saw are usually used to cut open the skull. Surgery is then performed on the injured part of the brain, and the part of the bone taken from the skull is stored in a freezer and is then replaced after the individual recovers.

However, during extreme injury, the skull bone can be broken badly, and in such situations, broken pieces of the bone cannot be substituted and are discarded. Once the neurosurgeon carefully removes the damaged part of the skull, the dura mater (outermost membrane of the brain) is then sliced to expose the nucleus that underlies it. The neurosurgeon maintains the wound without bleeding until every hematoma or contusion is extracted. When the brain becomes badly swollen, certain neurosurgeons prefer not to remove the bone until the swelling reduces, which may take up to a few weeks. In such cases, the neurosurgeon may decide to install an intracranial pressure (ICP) monitor to keep track of the patient's condition. The patient is later admitted to the intensive care unit (ICU) for further treatment.

CRANIOPLASTY

Cranioplasty is the surgical reconstruction of a bone defect of the skull, prior to surgery performed on the patient. There are various forms of cranioplasty, but most of them involve preserving the contour of the skull with the original piece of the skull or restoring the skull with a personalized contoured graft made of materials, such as:

- Acrylic (prefabricated or customized)
- Titanium (plate or mesh)
- Synthetic bone substitute

Conventional forms of cranioplasty include peeling back five layers of the scalp to insert the bone residue or customized implant in the proper cranial location. The neurosurgeon takes back the three uppermost layers of the scalp for pericranial-onlay cranioplasty, a modern procedure, and places the bone or implant in between the third and fourth layers.

MEDICAL CARE FOR TRAUMATIC BRAIN INJURY SURGERIES

The management of TBI presents many challenges to neurosurgeons and intensivists involved in surgical procedures. Most patients with mild to serious head trauma are taken to the operation room straight from the emergency ward. In certain instances, surgery is performed to extract a large hematoma or contusion that greatly compresses the brain or raises the pressure inside the skull. Such patients are typically treated and monitored in the ICU following surgery.

To track the pressure in the brain cavity, a bolt or ICP control system can be mounted within the skull. This can be surgically extracted or eliminated if bleeding occurs inside the skull cavity. In extreme situations, where significant inflammation and weakened brain tissue is present, a section can be extracted surgically to allow space for live brain tissue.

The overall purpose of any surgical care is to reduce serious damage by allowing the brain to retain air supply and oxygen and to decrease inflammation and pain.

Emergency surgery may be required to reduce any damage to brain tissue.

BENEFITS OF SURGERY

The following complications can be resolved by surgery:

- **Removing clotted blood (hematomas).** Bleeding outside or within the brain may result in an accumulation of clotted blood (hematoma). This causes strain to the brain and destroys brain tissue.
- **Repairing skull fractures.** Surgery can be required to fix serious skull fractures or to remove skull fragments in the brain.
- **Bleeding in the brain.** Head injuries that cause damage to the brain may require surgery to stop the bleeding.
- **Opening a window in the skull.** Surgery may be used to alleviate pressure inside the skull by removing

accumulated spinal cerebral fluid or by opening a gap in the skull that offers more space for swelling tissue.

In some head injuries, contusions or hematomas may enlarge over the first few hours or days after the injury. The safest approach for the patient may be to remove the lesion before it enlarges and causes neurological damage.

References

1. Villines, Zawn. "What Is a Decompressive Craniectomy?" Medical News Today, October 20, 2017.
2. "Traumatic Brain Injury," Mayo Clinic, March 29, 2019.
3. "Traumatic Brain Injury," American Association of Neurological Surgeons, February 15, 2000.
4. "Cranioplasty," Johns Hopkins Medicine, June 6, 2014.

Chapter 11 | **Emergency Treatment Guidelines Improve Survival of People with Severe Head Injury**

A large study of more than 21,000 people found that training emergency medical services (EMS) agencies to implement prehospital guidelines for traumatic brain injury (TBI) may help improve survival in patients with severe head trauma. The findings were published in *JAMA Surgery*, and the study was supported by the National Institute of Neurological Disorders and Stroke (NINDS), part of the National Institutes of Health (NIH).

"This demonstrates the significance of conducting studies in real-world settings and brings a strong evidence base to the guidelines," said Patrick Bellgowan, Ph.D., program director at NINDS. "It suggests we can systematically increase the chances of saving the lives of thousands of people who suffer severe traumatic brain injuries."

Based on scores of observational studies, guidelines for prehospital management of TBI that were developed in 2000, and updated in 2007, focused on preventing low oxygen, low blood pressure, and hyperventilation in people with head injury. Collectively, the

This chapter includes text excerpted from "Emergency Treatment Guidelines Improve Survival of People with Severe Head Injury," National Institute of Neurological Disorders and Stroke (NINDS), May 8, 2019.

studies suggested that controlling those factors before patients arrived at the hospital could improve survival, but actual adherence to the guidelines had not been examined.

The Excellence in Prehospital Injury Care (EPIC) Study, led by Daniel Spaite, M.D., professor of emergency medicine at the University of Arizona in Tucson, trained EMS agencies across Arizona in the TBI guidelines and compared patient outcomes before and after the guideline implementation. All patients in the study experienced head injury with loss of consciousness. This public-health initiative was a collaboration between the university and the Arizona Department of Health Services (ADHS). The EPIC study is the first time that the guidelines were assessed in real-world conditions.

The results showed that implementing the guidelines did not affect overall survival of the entire group, which included patients who had moderate, severe, and critical injuries. However, further analysis revealed that the guidelines helped double the survival rate of people with severe TBI and triple the survival rate in severe TBI patients who had to have a breathing tube inserted by EMS personnel. The guidelines were also associated with an overall increase in survival to hospital admission.

"We found a therapeutic sweet spot and showed that the guidelines had an enormous impact on people with severe TBI. The guidelines did not make a difference in the moderate TBI group because those individuals would most likely have survived anyway and, unfortunately, the extent of injuries sustained in many critical patients was too extreme to overcome," said Dr. Spaite.

Bentley Bobrow, M.D., professor of emergency medicine at the University of Arizona and co-principal investigator for the study said, "It was exciting to see such dramatic outcomes resulting from a simple two-hour training session with EMS personnel."

Part 3 | Conditions Associated with Traumatic Brain Injury

Chapter 12 | **Alzheimer Disease, Dementia, and Traumatic Brain Injury**

ALZHEIMER DISEASE

Alzheimer disease (AD) is a progressive disorder that causes brain cells to degenerate and die. This disorder is the most prevalent form of dementia—a gradual deterioration in thinking, behavioral, and social abilities that disrupts a person's individual capacity to work.

Forgetting recent events or conversations are the usual early symptoms of this disorder. A person with AD will develop severe memory impairment as the disease progresses and will lose the ability to handle daily tasks. In advanced stages, the patient suffers complications from severe loss of brain function—such as dehydration, malnutrition, or infections, which may result in death.

Alzheimer disease medications may temporarily improve symptoms or slow the progress of the disorder. These treatments can sometimes help people with AD in maximizing functionality and maintaining independence for a period of time. Different programs and services can help support people with AD and their caregivers.

There is no treatment that cures AD or that alters the disease process in the brain. The largest established contributing factor is increasing age, as the majority of those with Alzheimer are over 65 years of age. However, Alzheimer is not just an old-age illness; the younger-onset AD (also known as "early-onset Alzheimer") has been detected in around 200,000 Americans under 65 years of age.

"Alzheimer Disease, Dementia, and Traumatic Brain Injury," © 2020 Omnigraphics. Reviewed May 2020.

TRAUMATIC BRAIN INJURY: A RISK FACTOR FOR ALZHEIMER DISEASE AND DEMENTIA

Severe traumatic brain injury (TBI) has been shown to increase levels of beta-amyloid protein within hours after injury. Dementia is characterized by deposits of tau protein.

Head injuries may play a potential role in problems ranging from mild cognitive impairments to full-blown dementia, including Alzheimer disease.

While there is minimal and clear proof of a correlation between moderate concussions and dementia, researches have shown that medium to a serious head injury can dramatically increase the risk of dementia.

Most studies and researches focus on autopsy and imaging, showing consistent pathology linked to different dementia types.

Possible explanations for the association between head trauma and dementia include the disruption of neurometabolic processes. This can occur due to rotational and shear forces that can destroy axons and trigger cytoskeletal injury. That may indicate progressive cell death and amyloid-beta plaque formation in the surrounding areas. Although proof of increased neurofibrillary tangles after a single TBI is not as strong, case reports of increased tangles have been recorded one year or more after mild-to-extreme TBI.

For brain-injured individuals, the nature of dementia differs considerably by type and location of head injury along with the characteristics of the individual before the head injury.

Many forms of dementia, such as AD, gradually worsens, though dementia from head injury does not get worse over time. The change usually takes months or years and is slow and gradual.

Mild Traumatic Injuries Tied to Alzheimer and Dementia

Evidence has linked mild-to-serious TBIs over the last 30 years to an increased risk of developing AD or another dementia, years after the first-head injury.

- Statistics indicate that elderly people with a history of mild TBI were 2.3 times more likely to experience AD than elders with no history of a head injury; while those with a history of extreme TBI were 4.5 times more likely to develop it.

- There is little data to show that one minor TBI raises the likelihood of dementia. However, research shows that repetitive minor traumatic brain effects such as those that may arise in sports including American soccer, football, hockey, and baseball, could be linked with a higher likelihood of chronic traumatic encephalopathy (CTE), a type of dementia.
- Not everyone sustaining a head injury experience dementia. Minor traumatic brain damage, commonly known as a "concussion," does not cause unconsciousness.

Mild traumatic brain injury symptoms may include:
- Inability to recall the origin of the accident or incidents happening just preceding or up to 24 hours after it happened.
- Confusion and disorientation
- Difficulty remembering new information
- Headache
- Dizziness
- Blurry vision
- Nausea and vomiting
- Ringing in the ears
- Trouble speaking coherently
- Changes in emotions or sleep patterns

MEDICATIONS FOR DEMENTIA AFTER A HEAD INJURY

There are no officially licensed drugs by the U.S. Food and Drug Administration (FDA) explicitly for managing dementia in individuals who have suffered a serious brain injury. Individuals suffering from brain injury may need treatment to relieve symptoms such as depression, mania, paranoia, impulsivity-aggression, irritability, mood fluctuations, anxiety, apathy, or focus impairments. Drug treatments can also ease headaches.

Psychotropic or psychoactive drugs are the labeled medicines used to relieve these effects. These drugs are believed to help dampen the behavior of brain areas when there is too much stimulation and to better regulate the operation of brain regions involved in perception, behavior, attitude management, and impulse control. Head-injured people are more prone to side effects of these drugs. Frequent adjustment of doses and schedules may be required to find out the best regimen. The same drugs are used to treat patients affected by dementia, either due to head injury or other diseases.

References

1. "Dementia in Head Injury," WebMD, October 16, 2018.
2. Vitelli, Romeo. "Can Traumatic Brain Injury Lead to Alzheimer's Disease?" Psychology Today, February 27, 2018.
3. "Traumatic Brain Injury (TBI)," Alzheimer's Association, March 23, 2016.

Chapter 13 | **Depression and Traumatic Brain Injury**

Although depression is one of several potential psychiatric illnesses that may be common following TBI, the extent to which depression contributes to long-term disability following traumatic brain injury (TBI) is not known. Major depression may be triggered by physical or emotional distress, and it can deplete the mental energy and motivation needed for both recovering from the depression itself and adapting to the physical, social, and emotional consequences of trauma with brain injury. Depression may be masked by other deficits after head injury, such as cognitive changes and flat affect, which may be blamed for lack of progress in posttrauma treatment but actually reflect underlying depression. Clinicians, caregivers, and patients lack formal evidence to guide the timing of depression screening, which tools to use for screening and assessment, treatment choices, and assessment of treatment success.

IMPORTANCE OF DEPRESSION

Depression is defined by criteria that likely circumscribe a heterogeneous set of illnesses. While no single feature is seen in all depressed patients, common features include sadness, persistent negative thoughts, apathy, lack of energy, cognitive distortions, nihilism, and inability to enjoy normal events in life. Especially,

This chapter includes text excerpted from "Traumatic Brain Injury and Depression," Agency for Healthcare Research and Quality (AHRQ), U.S. Department of Health and Human Services (HHS), April 2011. Reviewed May 2020.

in a first episode, individuals and families may not recognize the changes as part of an illness, making identification and self-reporting of the condition challenging. Active screening is essential to recognition, treatment, and prevention of recurrence.

The most salient consequence of depression is suicide. Suicide is usually impulsive and extremely difficult to predict and prevent. At least half of suicides occur in the context of a mood disorder. Depression reduces quality of life (QOL), impairs ability to function in social and work roles, and causes self-doubt and difficulty taking action, all of which can delay recovery from TBI. The *Diagnostic and Statistical Manual for Mental Disorders, Fourth Edition,* (DSM-IV-TR) defines the illness in terms of physiologic disturbances of sleep, appetite, attention and concentration, motor activity and energy, and of psychological losses of interest in normal activities, hope, and self-worth while ruminating with excessive sadness, guilt, and suicidal thoughts.

The disturbances may also occur following TBI due to other circumstances, such as pain that disrupts sleep, which may mask the recognition that the sleep disturbance is also a part of a burgeoning depression. Depression may be financially costly in undermining physical therapy efforts, treatment compliance in general, and rehabilitation planning and efforts. The need for systematic evaluation of the prevalence and consequences of depression following TBI is imperative, given the potential for mitigating suicide and unnecessary disability.

IMPORTANCE OF TRAUMATIC BRAIN INJURY

Traumatic brain injury occurs when external force from an event such as a fall, sports injury, assault, motor vehicle accident, or explosive blast injures the brain and causes loss of consciousness or loss of memory. TBI can result from direct impact to the head as well as from rapid acceleration or deceleration of brain tissue, which injures the brain by internal impact with the skull. Both mechanisms can cause tissue damage, swelling, inflammation, and internal bleeding.

Traumatic brain injury is responsible for roughly 1.2 million emergency department visits each year, with 1 in 4 patients requiring hospitalization. Because most estimates of TBI rates are based on hospital use, some individuals with TBI are not counted because they do not seek care at all, or they seek care in other settings. The Centers for Disease Control and Prevention (CDC) estimates that up to 75 percent of TBIs are mild in terms of duration of loss of consciousness and other immediate symptoms, meaning substantial underestimation of the number of individuals affected is likely.

Nonetheless, estimates of direct and indirect costs associated with TBI exceed $56 billion each year. Among individuals who sustain a TBI, approximately 50,000 die each year of their injuries and 80,000 to 90,000 will have a long-term disability. More than 5 million survivors of TBI live with chronic disability.

Military service carries a high risk of TBI. Traumatic brain injury is more common in the military than in civilian populations, even in peacetime. Advances in body protection systems have resulted in fewer deaths and a concomitant rise in TBI that is more often moderate to severe than mild. The military confirms that more than 50,000 veterans who have returned from current theatres have blast-related TBI. As many as 30 percent of those with any injury on active duty have sustained a TBI. Because TBI is common, serious, and has high personal and economic costs, understanding potential consequences of injury is crucial.

RELATIONSHIP BETWEEN TRAUMATIC BRAIN INJURY AND DEPRESSION

TBIs are associated with a range of short- and long-term outcomes, including physical, cognitive, behavioral, and emotional impairment. Prior estimates, not derived systematically, of depression among individuals with TBI range widely, from 15 to 77 percent. Depression associated with TBI can manifest shortly after injury or well into the future. In their review of rehabilitation for TBI patients, Gordon and colleagues identified 74 studies of psychiatric functioning after TBI. Their assessment was that TBI is associated with high rates of depression—more than half of cases—and other DSM Axis I and Axis II conditions. Depression was noted to coexist with other psychiatric conditions, including addiction or anxiety.

Comorbid psychiatric conditions with depression may complicate screening, diagnosis, and management of depression in multiple ways, including masking depression so it remains undiagnosed or affects the individual's follow through or adherence to treatment. It is likely that such comorbid conditions complicate treatment response and recovery just as they do in non-TBI depressed patients. However, no systematic examination of this question has been done to date.

Triggers for depression after TBI may include biological, psychological, and social factors, and in the post-TBI population, greater attention is often given to biological factors because of the direct injury to the brain. However, many post-TBI patients do not demonstrate radiological or pathological evidence of brain injury, and in the context of current understanding of depression as a biopsychosocial entity, researchers and clinicians generally consider all depression to have a complex etiologic basis. Just as in the non-TBI population, the psychological impact of decreased occupational and functional abilities and its potential to affect the likelihood of becoming depressed should not be overlooked.

Chapter 14 | **Hypertension and Severe Traumatic Brain Injury**

HYPERTENSION

High blood pressure, also known as "hypertension," is a common condition where the force exerted by blood in the body against the walls of the arteries is high. This may eventually cause health problems and even heart diseases. The amount of blood pumped by the heart and amount of resistance of blood flow into the arteries determine the pressure of blood. While the arteries are narrowed and the heart pumps blood, a significant rise in the blood pressure can be seen.

Intracranial hypertension is a condition involving elevated pressure in the areas surrounding the brain and spinal cord. Many disorders may trigger persistent intracranial hypertension, including some medications, such as tetracycline, blood clot in the brain, inadequate consumption of vitamin A, or brain tumor.

HYPERTENSION AND TRAUMATIC BRAIN INJURY

Traumatic brain injury (TBI) is a significant public-health problem, with serious TBI leading to a substantial amount of fatalities and disabilities worldwide. Late hypertension after serious TBI was related to poor outcomes; therefore, guidelines recommend early and effective management of hypertension after TBI. Systemic hypertension and tachycardia in the acute stage of TBI are often observed.

High blood pressure, tachycardia, enhanced cardiac activity, regular or reduced peripheral vascular resistance, and elevated circulating catecholamines commonly distinguish arterial hypertension that develops following serious head injury.

COMPLICATIONS DUE TO HYPERTENSION

When high blood pressure causes pressure on the artery walls, it is bound to damage blood vessels, as well as the organs in the body. The longer the blood pressure stays uncontrolled, the greater the risk.

The complications in the human body due to high blood pressure include:

- **Heart attack or stroke**. The arteries start to harden and thicken due to high blood pressure. This condition, known as "atherosclerosis," can cause hardening and thickening of the arteries leading to a heart attack, stroke, or other complications. The heart tends to work harder to pump blood against the higher pressure in vessels. The pumping chamber of the heart starts to thicken due to this (left ventricular hypertrophy) and eventually makes it harder to pump blood. This can lead to end-stage heart failure.
- **Aneurysm**. Increased blood pressure may weaken and bulge the blood vessels, causing an aneurysm. A ruptured aneurysm may be life-threatening.
- **Kidney issues**. The blood vessels in the kidneys start to weaken and narrow, preventing these organs from functioning normally.
- **Vision problem**. The blood vessels in the eyes start to thicken, narrow, and tear, resulting in vision loss.
- **Metabolic syndrome**. The disorder is a collection of physiological anomalies in the body, including high waist circumference; elevated triglycerides; low high-density lipoprotein (HDL)—"good" cholesterol; high blood pressure, and high rates of insulin. Such

disorders result in a higher risk of contracting diabetes, cardiac failure, and stroke.

- **Trouble with memory or understanding.** Uncontrolled hypertension will also impair the ability to perceive, recall, and understand. Memory issues or conceptions of perception are more prevalent in individuals with elevated blood pressure.
- **Dementia.** Narrowed or blocked arteries may limit blood flow to the brain, resulting in some form of dementia (vascular dementia). A stroke that inhibits the flow of blood to the brain may also cause vascular dementia.

SYMPTOMS OF HYPERTENSION

High blood pressure can be present over the years without any symptoms, readings can reach dangerously high levels, and can continue to damage the blood vessels and heart. Heart attack, stroke, and serious health problems can occur from uncontrolled hypertension. High blood pressure symptoms in some people include:

- Bleeding from nose
- Shortness in breath
- Frequently occurring severe headaches
- Fatigue or feeling tired
- Confusion on decision making
- Vision problems
- Chest pain
- Irregular heartbeat
- Blood in the urine
- Pounding in your chest, neck, or ears

These symptoms are not specific and they usually do not occur until hypertension has reached a severe or a life-threatening stage.

MANAGEMENT OF HYPERTENSION

Propranolol and hydralazine are the two drugs used in the management of hypertension in head-injured patients. Both drugs effectively normalized blood pressure. According to experiments and statistics, as propranolol normalizes blood pressure and the underlying hemodynamic abnormalities, it appears to be a useful antihypertensive drug for severely head-injured patients.

References
1. "High Blood Pressure (Hypertension)," Mayoclinic, May 12, 2018.
2. Shiozaki, Tadahiko. "Hypertension and Head Injury," Researchgate, February 24, 2014.
3. "Symptoms of High Blood pressure," WebMD, May 23, 2018.

Chapter 15 | **Parkinson Disease and Traumatic Brain Injury**

PARKINSON DISEASE

Parkinson disease (PD) is a chronic condition that affects movements. This progressive nervous system disorder occurs when nerve cells or neurons in the brain that controls movement become impaired and/or die. Men have 50 percent more chances of being affected by this nervous disorder. For Parkinson, one strong risk factor is age. While most people with Parkinson first develop this disease after 60 years of age, around 5 to 10 percent of people with Parkinson have an "early-onset" disorder that starts before 50 years of age. Early-onset manifestations of Parkinson are hereditary often but not necessarily, although certain variants have been related to particular gene mutations.

PARKINSON DISEASE AND TRAUMATIC BRAIN INJURY

Studies show that traumatic brain injury (TBI) (typically secondary to car accidents, falls, or sports-related injuries) is associated with an increased risk of Parkinson disease (PD). While the link between them is already known, studies further support it by comparing the history of head trauma or brain injury between groups of people with and without Parkinson.

Dopamine is an important chemical produced by neurons in the brain. When these neurons die or become impaired due to a head injury, the production of dopamine is affected, which leads to movement problems. Norepinephrine is a chemical messenger of the nervous system that controls body functions, such as heart rate and blood pressure. Individuals affected by severe head trauma or injury lose the nerve endings that produce this norepinephrine. The loss of norepinephrine causes fatigue, a sudden drop in blood pressure while trying to stand up, decreased movement of food through the digestive tract, and even irregular blood pressure. These are a few nonmovement features of PD.

Traumatic brain injury can destroy the neural tissue and allow cellular breakdown products to be extracted from damaged cells in the surrounding environment. The cellular breakdown products will then act on healthy adjacent cells and facilitate aggregation of the intracellular alpha-synuclein. Men in the United States contribute for more TBIs and are almost twice as likely to be affected with PD. While the gender variations are not well known, some researches say that estrogen could be responsible for the neuroprotection and milder symptoms observed in women at the onset of PD.

Research shows that veterans with a history of TBI had a 56 percent greater chance of experiencing PD later in life and that this probability grows with increased intensity of TBI. Brain injury due to bomb blasts is the leading cause of injuries in veterans, similar to TBIs in athletes, such as football players and boxers. They are more inclined to suffer from PD compared to the general population. Studies show that microvascular nerve cell damage, neuroinflammation, and increased levels of harmful oxidative stress occur hours and days even after a mild blast-induced brain injury.

SIGNS AND SYMPTOMS

The symptoms start gradually, sometimes with a barely noticeable tremor in the hand, followed by stiffness or slowing of movement.

A few common Parkinson signs and symptoms may include:

- **Tremor.** A tremor (shaking) usually begins in the limbs, often in the hand or fingers. The patient may rub the thumb and forefinger back-and-forth, known as a "pill-rolling tremor." The hand may also start shaking when it is at rest.

- **Slowed movement (bradykinesia).** Parkinson disease may slow down body movement, making simple tasks difficult and time-consuming. Steps taken may become shorter when walking and the feet may start to drag. It may be difficult to get out of a chair.
- **Rigid muscles.** Muscle stiffness may occur in any part of the body and the stiff muscles can be painful and limit the range of motion.
- **Impaired posture and balance.** The person's posture may become stooped, or the person may develop balance problems as a result of Parkinson disease.
- **Loss of automatic movements.** Reduced ability to perform unconscious movements such as smiling, blinking, or swinging the arms when walking.
- **Speech changes.** The patient may speak softly, quickly, slur, or hesitate before talking. Speech may not have the usual inflections and can be monotonous.
- **Writing changes.** It may become hard to write, and the writing may appear small.

TREATING PARKINSON DISEASE AFTER HEAD INJURY

There is currently no cure for Parkinson. However, it is possible to treat the symptoms through physical therapy and medications.

Physical Therapy

Physical therapy (PT) helps in the improvement of muscle strength and control, helping to reduce tremors and dystonia, both of which are common symptoms of Parkinson disease. PT exercises can activate the brain's neuroplasticity and strengthen the neural signals sent to the muscles. Orthotic braces or weights are fixed to keep the affected muscle stable and to stop tremors.

Speech Therapy

Parkinson is known for causing hand tremors and slowed movement. It can also cause speech problems as tremors can affect a person's voice box or throat muscles making it difficult to swallow or talk. To treat this, the speech therapists are trained in an intensive therapy technique called "Lee Silverman Voice Treatment (LSVT)" that is specifically designed for Parkinson patients. This involves 16 sessions in a month, which can greatly improve a person's quality of life (QOL).

Medications

Medications to treat Parkinson disease mostly focus on increasing the dopamine levels in the brain. Some common medications prescribed includes:

- **Carbidopa-levodopa**, a naturally occurring chemical that converts into dopamine while entering the brain
- **Dopamine agonists**, drugs that release a chemical to imitate the effects of dopamine in the brain
- **Amantadine**, an antiviral drug that improves muscle control and reduces stiffness

Deep Brain Stimulation

Doctors might recommend surgical interventions to treat tremors and other symptoms in severe parkinsonism cases. The most common clinical procedure for tremors is deep brain stimulation (DBS). This requires electrodes that are surgically inserted to transmit high-frequency impulses to the thalamus (the part that controls involuntary movements). The electric impulses are transmitted from a tiny unit, identical to a pacemaker, that is positioned in the chest of the person under the skin. As the signal reaches the thalamus, the tremors are disabled.

References

1. "Parkinson's Disease," Mayoclinic, June 30, 2018.
2. Delic, Vedad; Beck, Kevin D; Pang, Kevin C. H; Citron, Bruce A. "Biological Links between Traumatic Brain Injury and Parkinson's disease," April 7, 2020.

3. "Ask the MD: Head Trauma and Parkinson's Disease," The Michael J. Fox Foundation, June 17, 2016.
4. "Can Head Injury Cause Parkinson's Disease? Understanding the Link Between TBI and Parkinsonism," Flintrehab, February 13, 2020.

Chapter 16 | Polytrauma and Traumatic Brain Injury

Traumatic brain injury (TBI) is an injury or blow to the head by an external force, disrupting the normal brain functionalities. The brain becomes particularly susceptible to injury as a consequence of crashes, collisions involving a motor vehicle, or assaults.

The medical term 'polytrauma' is defined as a state involving injury to the organs of the body leading to metabolic changes in the human system. In short, polytrauma is a result of injuries to multiple body parts and organs. It is frequently referred to as a combination of:

- Two major system injuries and one limb injury
- One major system injury and two limb injuries
- One major system injury along with an open grade III skeletal injury
- Unstable pelvic fracture with associated visceral injury

Polytrauma can result in prolonged hospitalization and, in some cases, it can even lead to death. Deaths with polytrauma arise in a patterned way, which may be assumed to be three points. Severe neurological or vascular injuries, the first point is seen within minutes, so immediate medical treatments can barely improve the outcome. The second point occurs during the "golden hour." It may be attributed to an intracranial hematoma, severe abdominal, or thoracic damage. This is the need with the Specialized Emergency

Life Support (ATLS) approach becoming the main target of the action. After days or weeks, the third phase emerges due to sepsis or multiple organ failure.

POLYTRAUMA AND TRAUMATIC BRAIN INJURY

When TBI is combined with a severe secondary injury (amputation, burns, fractures), the subsequent "polytrauma" can have severe consequences that compound those found in TBI alone. Polytrauma is not always a result of blast-related events. Disabling conditions such as amputation, burns, spinal cord injury (SCI), auditory and visual damage, and other medical conditions, are the common causes for polytrauma. Polytrauma associated with traumatic brain injury (TBI) is characterized as a cumulative brain injury and it affects one or more areas of the body or organ systems that contribute to physical, cognitive, and psychosocial disability.

POLYTRAUMA AND TBI IN VETERANS

In modern military operations, substantial developments in safety equipment and medical technologies have improved the recovery levels of all service members suffering serious traumatic injuries, or polytrauma. Polytrauma treatment is a patient-centered, interdisciplinary strategy that deals with the wounded victim and her or his families to resolve all facets of the accident as it impacts the life of the individual.

In the military conflicts, polytrauma is primarily caused by proximity to an explosive event. Advances in military medicine and protective gear have helped save lives. Rehabilitation works to optimize recovery and facilitate return to independent living and higher quality of life (QOL). As a consequence, TBI-accompanied polytrauma presents a specific challenge for emergency medicine, especially to those familiar with the austere conditions faced in military operating theaters and en-route treatment logistics. Veterans and military veterans with polytrauma need a high degree of integration and management of health treatment and other support resources because of the extent and scope of their injuries.

COMPLICATIONS OF POLYTRAUMA AND TBI

Managing a head injury patient with several other conditions poses one of the most complex and challenging surgical situations of serious trauma treatment. This is attributed in part to the assumption that care of certain conditions such as orthopedic, spinal, and craniofacial disorders, has the ability to cause neurological results worse. The possible complication is not inherently specifically linked to the main treatment or scheduling of operation but rather to the reality that subsequent intervention and probable blood loss and likely associated hypotension or hypoxia will negatively impact a damaged brain. A single episode of hypotension or hypoxia can adversely affect the outcome of all headache severities.

REHABILITATION CARE FOR POLYTRAUMA AND TBI

The polytrauma system of care (PSC) offers an integrated, organized, and systematic process of care for polytrauma/brain injury patients. Such facilities vary from comprehensive medical care to therapeutic and ambulatory initiatives intended to treat all facets of injury. The programs are provided across the country to civilians, veterans, their military families and have been active in the primary treatment of hundreds of thousands of wounded combat troops. Assistive technology labs, transitional rehabilitation programs, telehealth services, drivers' training programs, and emerging consciousness programs are the few regular types of programs to help patients affected by polytrauma and TBI.

References

1. Schuster, James M. "Head Injuries in Polytrauma Patients," Springlink, February 16, 2013.
2. "Polytrauma/TBI System of Care," U.S. Department of Veteran Affairs, March 4, 2019.
3. Tortella, Frank C.; Leung, Lai Yee. "Traumatic Brain Injury and Polytrauma in Theaters of Combat," Shock Society, March 30, 2020.
4. "Rehabilitation Care of Combat Related TBI: Veterans Health Administration Polytrauma System of Care," Springer Nature Switzerland AG, July 11, 2013.

Chapter 17 | **PTSD and Traumatic Brain Injury**

Traumatic brain injury (TBI) occurs from a sudden blow or jolt to the head. Brain injury often occurs during some type of trauma such as an accident, blast, or a fall. Often when people refer to TBI, they are mistakenly talking about the symptoms that occur following a TBI. Actually, a TBI is the injury, not the symptoms.

HOW SERIOUS IS MY INJURY?

A TBI is basically the same thing as a concussion. A TBI can be mild, moderate, or severe. These terms tell you the nature of the injury itself. They do not tell you what symptoms you may have or how severe the symptoms will be.

A TBI can occur even when there is no direct contact to the head. For example, when a person suffers whiplash, the brain may be shaken within the skull. This damage can cause bleeding between the brain and skull. Bruises can form where the brain hits the skull. Like bruises on other parts of the body, for mild injuries these will heal with time.

About 80 percent of all TBIs in civilians are mild (mTBI). Most people who have an mTBI will be back to normal by three months without any special treatment. Even patients with moderate or severe TBI can make remarkable recoveries.

The length of time that a person is unconscious (knocked out) is one way to measure how severe the injury was. If you were not knocked out at all or if you were out for less than 30 minutes, your TBI

This chapter includes text excerpted from "Traumatic Brain Injury and PTSD," National Center for Posttraumatic Stress Disorder (NCPTSD), U.S. Department of Veterans Affairs (VA), October 17, 2019.

was most likely minor or mild. If you were knocked out for more than 30 minutes but less than six hours, your TBI was most likely moderate.

WHAT ARE THE COMMON SYMPTOMS FOLLOWING A TRAUMATIC BRAIN INJURY?

Symptoms that result from TBI are known as "postconcussion syndrome" (PCS). Few people will have all of the symptoms, but even one or two of the symptoms can be unpleasant. PCS makes it hard to work, get along at home, or relax. In the days, weeks, and months following a TBI the most common symptoms are:

Physical
- Headache
- Feeling dizzy
- Being tired
- Trouble sleeping
- Vision problems
- Feeling bothered by noise and light

Cognitive (Mental)
- Memory problems
- Trouble staying focused
- Poor judgment and acting without thinking
- Being slowed down
- Trouble putting thoughts into words

Emotional (Feelings)
- Depression
- Anger outbursts and quick to anger
- Anxiety (fear, worry, or feeling nervous)
- Personality changes

These symptoms are part of the normal process of getting better. They are not signs of lasting brain damage. These symptoms are to be expected and are not a cause for concern or worry. More serious symptoms include severe forms of those listed above, decreased response to standard treatments, and seizures.

DO I HAVE THE SYMPTOMS THAT FOLLOW A TBI OR PTSD— OR BOTH?

You may notice that many of the symptoms that follow a TBI overlap with the common reactions after trauma. Because TBI is caused by trauma and there is symptom overlap, it can be hard to tell what the underlying problem is. In addition, many people who get a TBI also develop posttraumatic stress disorder (PTSD).

It is important to be assessed because:

- People with TBI should not use some medications.
- No matter how mild or severe the injury itself was, the effects could be serious.

Although TBI screens are used, a screen is not used to diagnose TBI. Even if your TBI screen is positive, that does not mean that you have a TBI. It means that you should be assessed further.

Diagnosing a TBI is hard because there may not be any physical signs of injury. Details of the trauma may be hard to pin down. Sometimes right after the injury the effects are so brief that they are not noticed. You may go to the doctor sometime later when details of the injury are not as clear. TBI can occur in confused times of crisis, such as combat. In the heat of events the injury may be ignored. Many of the symptoms that can result from a TBI are the same as the symptoms of PTSD. For these reasons, the best way to diagnose a TBI is an interview by a skilled clinician.

ARE THERE EFFECTIVE TREATMENTS?

Many people recover from TBI without any formal treatment. Problems that linger may clear up in a few weeks. You may notice some problems more as you return to your normal routine. For example, you may not realize that you get tired more quickly until you return to your regular chores, work, or school. Even so, people usually get better after a head injury, not worse. Professional

treatment for the symptoms that follow TBI usually involves rehabilitation to improve functioning.

The good news is that effective treatments for PTSD also work
well for those who have suffered mTBI. This includes two forms
of therapy: Cognitive Processing Therapy (CPT) and Prolonged
Exposure (PE).

WHAT CAN I DO TO COPE?

The best way to deal with symptoms following TBI is to go back
slowly to your normal routine, a little at a time. How much time
you spend at work, with family, with others, or exercising depends
on what feels comfortable. Pace yourself, and be sure to get all the
rest you need. Avoiding alcohol and not taking any unnecessary
medications is a good idea, to help allow the brain to heal.

If your symptoms get worse, or if you notice new PCS symptoms,
this is a sign that you are pushing yourself too hard. Ignoring your
symptoms and trying to "tough it out" often make the symptoms
worse. Symptoms are your body's way of giving you information. A
broken bone or a torn muscle hurts so that you will not use it and
it has time to heal. PCS symptoms are your brain's way of telling
you that you need to rest it.

Research suggests that one week of relaxing at home and then a
week of slowly doing more after leaving the hospital is best for most
patients. Most patients who took this advice were back to normal
at work or school in 3 to 4 weeks. Most patients who were not told
what to do took 5 to 12 weeks to get back to their normal routine.
They also had more PCS symptoms than patients who returned
slowly to their routines.

Accept and Deal with the Stress of the Injury

Be aware that having a head injury adds more stress to your life,
not just bumps and bruises to your head. The trauma itself, being
in the hospital, and going back to work or school and normal routines are all things that add stress to most patients' lives. You may
have some trouble with work or school at first, and even though it
is normal, this may be stressful and frustrating.

Another main cause of stress after a TBI is worry about the symptoms you have. Thinking and worrying about your symptoms can make them seem worse. Doctors who treat TBI agree that the single most important factor in recovery is that you know what to expect and what to do about the symptoms. You should remember that the symptoms are a normal part of getting better. They will likely go away on their own.

Involve Family
Any level of TBI can disrupt families. Roles and responsibilities change when a family member is hurt. From the start, families need to be involved and informed about TBI. By supporting the family, patient outcomes can be improved and burnout prevented.

Return to School or Work Slowly
Returning to school or work is often the biggest challenge after TBI. This is because PCS symptoms can get in the way of meeting your work and school demands. For example, trouble focusing and memory problems may make it harder to learn new things in school. Or fatigue may limit your being able to handle work demands. Keep in mind when trying to return to work or school that the process will be slow. Do not expect yourself to perform right away as you did before your TBI. Instead, you should slowly resume responsibilities as you are able. Slowly increase your workload and hours. Only increase them when you feel fully ready.

TRAUMATIC BRAIN INJURY AND VETERANS
The conflicts in Afghanistan and Iraq (OEF/OIF) have resulted in increased numbers of Veterans who have TBI. The main causes of TBI in OEF/OIF Veterans are blasts, motor vehicle accidents, and gunshot wounds. The Department of Defense (DOD) and the Defense and Veteran's Brain Injury Center (DVBIC) estimate that 22 percent of all OEF/OIF combat wounds are brain injuries. This is compared to TBI in 12 percent of combat wounds that occurred in Vietnam.

Veterans seem to have symptoms for longer than civilians. Some studies show most will still have symptoms 18 to 24 months after the TBI. Also, many Veterans have more than one medical problem, including: PTSD, chronic pain, or substance abuse. From 60 to 80 percent of Servicemembers who are hurt in other ways by a blast may have a TBI. These other problems make it harder to get better from any single problem. Veterans should remember, though, that their TBI symptoms are likely to last only a limited time. With proper treatment and healthy behaviors, they are likely to improve.

The VA is working to make sure that TBI care is easy to access. The VA is using a TBI screening tool to begin the assessment process. The VA has put in place the Polytrauma System of Care (PSC) to treat Veterans with TBI who also have other injuries. Veterans with the most severe wounds are being treated at one of the 4 Polytrauma Rehabilitation Centers (PRCs) or one of the 21 Polytrauma Network Sites (PNS). Patients with less severe wounds may get treatment at local VA Medical Centers. No matter where a Veteran goes first, there is no "wrong door" for treatment.

Chapter 18 | **Vision Loss and Traumatic Brain Injury**

Traumatic brain injury (TBI) occurs when the brain is harmed by an external force, such as a violent blow to the head or an object penetrating the skull. More than 1.4 million Americans receive treatment for TBI every year, while millions more suffer mild brain injuries—such as a concussion—and do not seek medical treatment. TBI can disrupt normal brain functioning and produce sensory, cognitive, or physical impairments that may be temporary or permanent. Many people with a TBI, or even a mild head injury, experience problems with their eyes and vision.

Situations that cause TBI can also cause trauma to the eyes or vision system, resulting in such sight-threatening conditions as retinal detachment, vitreous hemorrhage, or optic nerve damage. In addition to injuring the eyes directly, however, TBI can also cause vision problems by damaging parts of the brain involved in processing visual input from the eyes, such as the occipital lobe. Vision involves not only seeing with the eyes, but also interpreting, making sense of, and developing appropriate responses to visual images. Vision accounts for around 85 percent of the sensory input that is processed by the brain, and it affects perception, cognition, learning, motor skills, and other systems in the body. As a result, vision problems related to TBI can have a significant impact on people's everyday activities and overall quality of life (QOL).

"Traumatic Brain Injury and Vision Loss," © 2017 Omnigraphics. Reviewed May 2020.

COMMON TYPES OF VISION PROBLEMS

An accident that injures the brain can also cause physical injury to the eyes and vision system. Some of the potentially serious injuries that create vision problems include the following:

- **Retinal detachment.** The retina is a thin layer of photoreactive cells at the back of the eye that turns light images into nerve impulses and sends them to the brain for processing. A violent blow to the head can cause the retina to tear loose from the back of the eye. Without prompt medical treatment, retinal detachment can result in permanent blindness.
- **Optic nerve damage.** When TBI causes swelling of the brain, the increased pressure within the skull can cut off blood circulation to the optic nerve. Damage to the optic nerve can disrupt the flow of visual input from the eyes to the brain, sometimes resulting in permanent vision loss.
- **Vitreous hemorrhage.** The vitreous is a clear, jelly-like substance that fills the rear portion of the eye and allows light to pass through to the retina. A brain injury can break blood vessels in the eye and allow blood to enter the vitreous. Although such hemorrhages can disrupt vision temporarily, most cases clear up over time without causing permanent damage.

SYMPTOMS OF VISION PROBLEMS

Many other vision problems associated with TBI occur due to damage to parts of the brain involved in processing visual signals from the eyes. The symptoms vary depending on the extent of the injury, the parts of the brain that are affected, and the patient's individual recovery process. Some of the symptoms of vision problems that commonly result from traumatic brain injuries include the following:

- Blurry vision
- Double vision
- Sensitivity to light
- Headaches when performing visual tasks

- Motion sickness, nausea, or vomiting when performing visual tasks
- Difficulty reading
- Difficulty with visual attention, concentration, comprehension, or memory
- Visual balance disorders
- Decreased peripheral vision or reduction of visual field
- Inability to maintain visual contact or focus
- Difficulty with eye movements, including the ability to: change focus from near to distant objects; track moving objects; shift gaze quickly from one object to another; and achieve the eye teaming or alignment required for binocular vision and depth perception

IMPACT OF VISION PROBLEMS

The vision symptoms experienced by people with TBI can affect many aspects of their daily lives, including the ability to work, go to school, drive a car, participate in recreational activities, and perform self-care tasks. Some of the difficulties caused by dysfunction in the brain's ability to process visual images include the following:

- **Difficulty with reading or close work.** Many people with TBI or concussion experience blurry near vision, which can make it hard to read or look at a computer screen. They may find it difficult to focus on near objects, or text may appear to move or jump around.
- **Struggles with pain or discomfort.** Swelling inside the skull often causes headaches, eye pain, and nausea or motion sickness when performing visual tasks.
- **Issues with movement or balance.** Many people with TBI have trouble tracking moving objects with their eyes or judging the relative location of objects in space. They may feel as if the floor is tilted, or they may become dizzy when they turn around or lean to the side.
- **Difficulty processing and understanding visual information.** Injury to the occipital lobe can make it difficult for the brain to make sense of images seen by

the eyes. People with TBI may find it difficult to scan visual information, focus visual attention on objects, or recall visual information.

- **Anxiety or irritability in certain environments.** Visual problems associated with TBI may cause people to feel uncomfortable or distressed when confronted with certain visual input such as bright lights, complex patterns, or rapid motion.
- **Struggles with loss of vision or visual field.** People with decreased vision, double vision, or visual field loss face a risk of physical harm from bumping into objects, being struck by objects, or tripping over objects.

TREATMENT OF VISION PROBLEMS

It is important to seek medical attention for any type of head injury that results in vision problems. Treatment for TBI-related vision problems depends on the type of problem and underlying cause. An optometrist or ophthalmologist can provide treatment for eye issues that can be corrected with surgery, patching, corrective eyeglasses, magnifying eyeglasses, or special lenses, such as prism lenses. Eye doctors who specialize in visual problems related to TBI, such as neuro-ophthalmologists, may be needed for more complex problems involving the brain's visual processing center. Occupational therapists, vision rehabilitation therapists, and low vision specialists can also provide exercises, training, and adaptive devices aimed at decreasing or eliminating TBI-related vision problems.

MANAGEMENT OF VISION PROBLEMS

People with TBI can also use a number of strategies to adapt or manage the associated vision problems. Some suggestions include the following:

- Take frequent breaks to give the eyes and brain a rest while reading, using a computer, watching television, or doing other vision-dependent activities.
- Use magnifying lenses or increase print size and contrast on computer screens to make things easier to see.

- Avoid bright, fluorescent, and flashing lights or other visual input that might prove irritating to the eyes or brain.
- Wear tinted sunglasses to reduce glare and use glare-reducing filters on computer screens.
- Reduce visual input and overload by decluttering your home and work environment.
- Use adaptive devices such as talking appliances, audio books, screen-reading software and apps, and mobility canes to help with reduced vision or vision loss.

References

1. "About Vision Problems Associated with Brain Injuries." Optometrists Network, 2017.
2. Metcalf, Eric. "Head Injuries Can Lead to Serious Vision Problems." Everyday Health, January 20, 2009.
3. Politzer, Thomas. "Introduction to Vision and Brain Injury." Neuro-Optometric Rehabilitation Association, n.d.
4. Powell, Janet M.; Weintraub, Alan; Dreer, Laura; Novack, Tom. "Vision Problems and Traumatic Brain Injury." Model Systems Knowledge Translation Center, 2014.

Chapter 19 | **Epilepsy Following Traumatic Brain Injury**

WHAT IS EPILEPSY?

Epilepsy is a disorder of the brain that causes seizures. These seizures are not caused by a temporary underlying medical condition such as a high fever.

Epilepsy can affect people in very different ways. This is because there are many causes and many different kinds of seizures. Some people may have multiple types of seizures or other medical conditions in addition to epilepsy. These factors play a major role in determining both the severity of the person's condition and the impact it has on her or his life.

The way a seizure looks depends on the type of seizure a person is experiencing. Some seizures can look like staring spells. Other seizures can cause a person to collapse, shake, and become unaware of what's going on around them.

Epilepsy can be caused by different conditions that affect a person's brain. Many times the cause is unknown. Some causes include:
- Stroke
- Brain tumor

This chapter contains text excerpted from the following sources: Text under the heading "What Is Epilepsy?" is excerpted from "Epilepsy Fast Facts," Centers for Disease Control and Prevention (CDC), July 31, 2018; Text beginning the heading "Effects of Traumatic Brain Injury" is excerpted from "Epilepsy Can Follow Traumatic Brain Injury," Centers for Disease Control and Prevention (CDC), July 10, 2019.

- Traumatic brain injury or head injury
- Central nervous system infection

A person with epilepsy is not contagious and cannot give epilepsy to another person.

EFFECTS OF TRAUMATIC BRAIN INJURY

A traumatic brain injury (TBI) can happen to anyone, especially young children and older adults. TBIs can range from mild (such as concussions) to severe, life-threatening injuries. They can cause changes in:
- Thinking and memory
- Sensations and balance
- Language, such as talking and understanding
- Emotions such as depression, anxiety, or aggression.

HOW TRAUMATIC BRAIN INJURY CAN CAUSE EPILEPSY

Epilepsy is a broad term used for a brain disorder that causes repeated seizures. There are many types of epilepsies and there are also many different kinds of seizures. TBIs can cause a seizure right after the injury happens or even months or years later. Researchers agree that the more severe the TBI, the greater the chance the person may develop epilepsy. Age and other medical conditions are also factors in whether or not a person may develop epilepsy after a TBI.

The terms posttraumatic epilepsy (PTE) and posttraumatic seizures (PTS) are both used to describe seizures that happen because of a TBI. In 2014, there were over 280,000 hospitalizations for TBI in the United States. A Centers for Disease Control and Prevention (CDC)-funded study found that among people 15 years of age and older hospitalized for TBI, about 1 in 10 developed epilepsy in the following 3 years.

If you or someone you care for has a head injury, here is what you need to know:
- Seek medical attention and share information about TBI signs and symptoms.

- Talk to the doctor about the risk of having seizures or developing epilepsy after a TBI.
- Learn to recognize the signs of a seizure. Sometimes it can be hard to tell. Some seizures cause a person to fall, cry out, shake or jerk, and become unaware of what is going on around them. Other seizures can make a person appear confused, make it hard for them to answer questions, twitch, or cause the person to feel like they taste, see, or smell something unusual.
- Learn first aid so you are prepared if someone has a seizure.

To prevent TBIs that may cause epilepsy, protect your brain from injury. For example:

- Use seat belts and properly installed car safety seats every time you drive or ride in a motor vehicle.
- Never drive while under the influence of alcohol or drugs.
- Wear a helmet when playing certain sports and riding bikes, horses, motorcycles, or all-terrain vehicles.
- Prevent falls, especially in older adults and young children.

Part 4 | Disability from Traumatic Brain Injury

Chapter 20 | **Understanding Disability**

Chapter Contents

Section 20.1 | **Disability and Health Overview**

This section includes text excerpted from "Disability and Health Overview," Centers for Disease Control and Prevention (CDC), September 4, 2019

WHAT IS DISABILITY?

A disability is any condition of the body or mind (impairment) that makes it more difficult for the person with the condition to do certain activities (activity limitation) and interact with the world around them (participation restrictions).

There are many types of disabilities, such as those that affect a person's:

- Vision
- Movement
- Thinking
- Remembering
- Learning
- Communicating
- Hearing
- Mental health
- Social relationships

Although people with disabilities sometimes refers to a single population, this is actually a diverse group of people with a wide range of needs. Two people with the same type of disability can be affected in very different ways. Some disabilities may be hidden or not easy to see.

According to the World Health Organization (WHO), disability has three dimensions:

- Impairment in a person's body structure or function, or mental functioning; examples of impairments include loss of a limb, loss of vision, or memory loss
- Activity limitation such as difficulty seeing, hearing, walking, or problem-solving

- Participation restrictions in normal daily activities such as working, engaging in social and recreational activities, and obtaining healthcare and preventive services

Disability can be:
- Related to conditions that are present at birth and may affect functions later in life, including cognition (memory, learning, and understanding), mobility (moving around in the environment), vision, hearing, behavior, and other areas. These conditions may be:
  - Disorders in single genes (for example, Duchenne muscular dystrophy (DMD))
  - Disorders of chromosomes (for example, Down syndrome)
  - The result of the mother's exposure during pregnancy to infections (for example, rubella) or substances, such as alcohol or cigarettes
- Associated with developmental conditions that become apparent during childhood (for example, autism spectrum disorder (ASD) and attention deficit hyperactivity disorder or ADHD)
- Related to an injury (for example, traumatic brain injury (TBI) or spinal cord injury)
- Associated with a longstanding condition (for example, diabetes), which can cause a disability such as vision loss, nerve damage, or limb loss
- Progressive (for example, muscular dystrophy), static (for example, limb loss), or intermittent (for example, some forms of multiple sclerosis)

WHAT IS IMPAIRMENT?

Impairment is an absence of or significant difference in a person's body structure or function, or mental functioning. For example, problems in the structure of the brain can result in difficulty with mental functions, or problems with the structure of the eyes or ears can result in difficulty with the functions of vision or hearing.

- **Structural impairments** are significant problems with an internal or external component of the body. Examples of these include a type of nerve damage that can result in multiple sclerosis (MS), or a complete loss of a body component, such as when a limb has been amputated.
- **Functional impairments** include the complete or partial loss of function of a body part. Examples of these include pain that does not go away or joints that no longer move easily.

WHAT IS THE DIFFERENCE BETWEEN ACTIVITY LIMITATION AND PARTICIPATION RESTRICTION?

The World Health Organization (WHO) published the *International Classification of Functioning, Disability, and Health* (*ICF*) in 2001. The *ICF* provides a standard language for classifying body function and structure, activity, participation levels, and conditions in the world around us that influence health. This description helps to assess the health, functioning, activities, and factors in the environment that either help or create barriers for people to fully participate in society.

According to the *ICF*:

- Activity is the execution of a task or action by an individual.
- Participation is a person's involvement in a life situation.

The *ICF* acknowledges that the distinction between these two categories is somewhat unclear and combines them, although basically, activities take place at a personal level and participation involves engagement in life roles such as employment, education, or relationships. Activity limitations and participation restrictions have to do with difficulties an individual experiences in performing tasks and engaging in social roles. Activities and participation can be made easier or more difficult as a result of environmental factors such as technology, support, and relationships, services, policies, or the beliefs of others.

The *ICF* includes the following in the categories of activities and participation:

- Learning and applying knowledge
- Managing tasks and demands
- Mobility (moving and maintaining body positions, handling and moving objects, moving around in the environment, moving around using transportation)
- Managing self-care tasks
- Managing domestic life
- Establishing and managing interpersonal relationships and interactions
- Engaging in major life areas (education, employment, managing money or finances)
- Engaging in community, social, and civic life

It is very important to improve the conditions in communities by providing accommodations that decrease or eliminate activity limitations and participation restrictions for people with disabilities, so they can participate in the roles and activities of everyday life.

Section 20.2 | Living with Physical Disability

This section includes text excerpted from "Disability and Health Information for People with Disabilities," Centers for Disease Control and Prevention (CDC), October 28, 2019.

Since the Americans with Disabilities Act (ADA) was enacted in 1990, many social barriers have been removed or reduced for people with disabilities. But, there is more work that needs to be done for people with disabilities to become more independent and involved in their world. Good health is important to be able to work, learn, and be engaged within a community.

HEALTHY LIVING

People with disabilities need healthcare and health programs for the same reasons anyone else does—to stay well, active, and to be a part of the community.

Having a disability does not mean a person is not healthy or that she or he cannot be healthy. Being healthy means the same thing for all of us—getting and staying well so we can lead full, active lives. That means having the tools and information to make healthy choices and knowing how to prevent illness.

SAFETY

People with disabilities can be at higher risk for injuries and abuse. It is important for parents and other family members to teach their loved ones how to stay safe and what to do if they feel threatened or have been hurt in any way.

ASSISTIVE TECHNOLOGY

Assistive technologies (ATs) are devices or equipment that can be used to help a person with a disability fully engage in life activities. ATs can help enhance functional independence and make daily living tasks easier through the use of aids that help a person travel, communicate with others, learn, work, and participate in social and recreational activities. An example of an assistive technology can be anything from a low-tech device, such as a magnifying glass, to a high tech device, such as a special computer that talks and helps someone communicate. Other examples are wheelchairs, walkers, and scooters, which are mobility aids that can be used by persons with physical disabilities.

SCHOOL

In order to help a child fully participate in school, plans can be developed around the child's specific needs. These plans, known as "504 plans," are used by general education students not eligible for special education services. By law, children may be eligible to have a 504 plan which lists accommodations related to a child's disability. The 504 plan accommodations may be needed to give the child an opportunity to perform at the same level as their peers. For example, a 504 plan may include your child's assistive technology needs, such as a tape recorder or keyboard for taking notes and a wheelchair-accessible environment.

A different plan is needed for children taking special education classes. An Individual Education Plan (IEP) is a legal document that tells the school its duties to your child.

TRANSITIONS

For some people with disabilities and their parents, change can be difficult. Planning ahead of time may make transitions easier for everyone.

Transitions occur at many stages of life. For example, the transition from teen years to adulthood can be especially challenging. There are many important decisions to make such as deciding whether to go to college, a vocational school, or enter the workforce. It is important to begin thinking about this transition in childhood, so that educational transition plans are put in place. Ideally, transition plans from teen years to adulthood are in place by 14 years of age, but no later than 16 years of age. This makes sure the person has the skills she or he needs to begin the next phase of life. This stage in life also involves transitioning one's healthcare services from pediatricians to physicians who primarily treat adults.

INDEPENDENT LIVING

Independent living means that a person lives in her or his own apartment or house and needs limited or no help from outside agencies. The person may not need any assistance or might need help with only complex issues, such as managing money, rather than day-to-day living skills. Whether an adult with disabilities continues to live at home or moves out into the community depends in large part on her or his ability to manage everyday tasks with little or no help. For example, can the person clean the house, cook, shop, and pay bills? Is she or he able to use public transportation? Many families prefer to start with some supported living arrangements and move towards increased independence.

FINDING SUPPORT

For many people with disabilities and those who care for them, daily life may not be easy. Disabilities affect the entire family. Meeting the complex needs of a person with a disability can put families under a great deal of stress—emotional, financial, and sometimes even physical.

However, finding resources, knowing what to expect, and planning for the future can greatly improve the overall quality of life (QOL). If you have a disability or care for someone who does, it might be helpful to talk with other people who can relate to your experience.

Find a Support Network

By finding support within your community, you can learn more about resources available to meet the needs of families and people with disabilities. This can help increase confidence, enhance QOL, and assist in meeting the needs of family members.

A national organization that focuses on the disability, such as Spina Bifida Association, that has a state or local branch, such as Spina Bifida Association in your state, might exist. State or local area Centers for Independent Living (CIL)could also be helpful. United Way offices may be able to point out resources. Look in the phone book or on the web for phone numbers and addresses.

Other ways to connect with other people include camps, organized activities, and sports for people with disabilities. In addition, there are online support groups and networks for people with many different types of disabilities.

Talk with a Mental-Health Professional

Psychologists, social workers, and counselors can help you deal with the challenges of living with or caring for someone with a disability. Talk to your primary care physician for a referral.

147

Chapter 21 | What Disabilities Can Result from a Traumatic Brain Injury?

Disabilities are typically related to changes and limitations in:
- Cognition
- Emotion and behavior control
- Communication
- Sensation
- Motor function

People who have had a traumatic brain injury (TBI) of any severity commonly have problems at first with cognition, which can include trouble remembering things, thinking of the right word, learning new information, problem-solving, concentrating, initiating activities, organizing, making decisions, and doing more than one thing at a time (multitasking).

Some people who have a TBI may have emotional or behavioral difficulties such as depression, apathy, anxiety, anger, confusion, sleep disruption, changes in controlling behavior, and mood swings. These difficulties may lead to impulsiveness and lack of self-control, violence, or inappropriate sexual activity.

This chapter includes text excerpted from "Brain Injuries: Prevention, Rehabilitation, and Community Living," Administration for Community Living (ACL), June 18, 2015. Reviewed May 2020.

Communicating with others can be a problem for those with TBI. Some may have difficulty with understanding, speaking, writing, and interpreting nonverbal signals, such as body language and the emotional cues of others. These problems can lead to miscommunication, confusion, and frustration for persons with TBI and for those who spend time with them.

Some people who have experienced a TBI have problems with vision and hand-eye coordination or movement. They may bump into or drop things, or feel unsteady.

Some people with TBI may need medicine to help them cope with the mental and physical-health problems they may experience. They are more likely to experience side effects from their medicine than those without TBI.

Chapter 22 | Victimization of People with Traumatic Brain Injury or Other Disabilities

WHAT IS VICTIMIZATION?

Victimization is harm caused on purpose. It is not an "accident" and can happen anywhere. While anyone can be victimized, people with disabilities are at greater risk for victimization than people without disabilities. This chapter provides a general overview of victimization and the risks to people with traumatic brain injury (TBI) and other disabilities.

WHAT DOES VICTIMIZATION INCLUDE?

- Physical violence with or without a weapon
- Sexual violence of any kind including rape
- Emotional abuse, including verbal attacks or being humiliated
- Neglect of personal needs for daily life, including medical care or equipment

This chapter includes text excerpted from "Victimization of Persons with Traumatic Brain Injury or Other Disabilities: A Fact Sheet for Friends and Families," Centers for Disease Control and Prevention (CDC), June 17, 2019.

HOW OFTEN DOES VICTIMIZATION OCCUR?

- In the United States, people with disabilities are 4 to 10 times more likely to be victimized than people without them.
- Children with disabilities are more than twice as likely to be victimized as children without them.

WHAT IS KNOWN ABOUT VICTIMIZATION?

- The two most common places for victimization are hospitals and at home.
- Victims usually know the person who harms them. They can be healthcare workers, intimate partners, or family members. More men than women cause harm to people with disabilities.

WHY ARE PEOPLE WITH A TRAUMATIC BRAIN INJURY AT RISK FOR VICTIMIZATION?

A TBI may cause problems that can increase risk. Known problems include:

- Difficulty understanding risky situations or avoiding risky persons
- Difficulty controlling one's temper which causes others to get angry
- Behavioral problems, such as drinking too much

WHAT CAN BE DONE TO HELP A FRIEND OR FAMILY MEMBER WHO IS BEING VICTIMIZED?

- Do not be afraid to voice your concern for their safety.
- Acknowledge that they are in a very difficult and scary situation.
- Be supportive.
- Do not be judgmental.
- Encourage them to talk to people who can provide help and guidance.

- Help them plan safety steps so that they will know what to do and how to reduce their risk of harm when they are being victimized.
- Remember that you cannot "rescue" them.

Chapter 23 | Support Services for People with Disabilities

Chapter Contents

Section 23.1 | Getting Help with My Medical Bills

This section includes text excerpted from "Financial Assistance and Support Services for People with Disabilities," USA.gov, December 12, 2019.

Below are the ways to find help from the government with medical bills and insurance options.

MEDICAID AND CHILDREN'S HEALTH INSURANCE PROGRAM HEALTHCARE FOR CHILDREN
What Help Is Available?

Medicaid and the Children's Health Insurance Program (CHIP) provides help with paying medical costs for children of families who cannot afford health insurance or do not get it through their work.

SOCIAL SECURITY AND MEDICARE
What Help Is Available?

Local Social Security Administration (SSA) offices help those on Social Security and Medicare find help. People over 65 years of age, people with disabilities under 65 years of age, and people with end-stage kidney disease are eligible for Medicare.

MEDICAID FOR ADULTS
What Help Is Available?

You may qualify for Medicaid, a joint federal and state program that helps with medical costs for some people with limited income from the Centers for Medicare and Medicaid Services (CMS).

Am I Eligible?

Each state has different rules about eligibility and applying for Medicaid for adults.

How Do I Apply?

Each state has different application requirements for Medicaid for adults. Call your state Medicaid program to see if you qualify and to learn how to apply.

HEALTH INSURANCE
THROUGH THE HEALTH INSURANCE MARKETPLACE
What Help Is Available?

HealthCare.gov helps you find insurance options, compare care, learn about preventive services, and more. If your employer does not offer insurance, you are self-employed, or you prefer to purchase your own insurance, you and your family can get health, dental, and vision insurance through the Health Insurance Marketplace.

Am I Eligible?

Everyone is eligible for health insurance through the Marketplace. You may also qualify for subsidies to help pay your premiums. If you have experienced certain life changes, such as loss of a job or childbirth, you may be eligible to make changes to your health insurance in a Special Enrollment Period (SEP).

How Do I Apply?

How you apply for a plan in the Health Insurance Marketplace depends on what plan you choose.

How Do I Complain or Where Do I Call for Additional Help?

Visit the Health Insurance Marketplace's top questions section for additional help with finding or applying for healthcare. To file a complaint, call 800-318-2596 (TTY: 855-889-4325).

IS THERE ANYTHING ELSE I NEED TO KNOW?

If you need more help getting or paying for medical care, try these resources:

- Contact your state or local social services agencies to find out if you qualify for any healthcare programs in your area.

- Community clinics offer free or low-cost medical services including prenatal care.
- Research institutes including the National Cancer Institute (NCI) and the National Institutes of Health (NIH) often list clinical trials and studies that are seeking participants for research on medications and certain medical conditions.
- Find out how you may be able to lower the cost of your prescription drugs and medical devices.
- Charity care programs help uninsured patients who cannot afford to pay their medical bills and do not qualify for government aid. The patient services department of your local hospital can help you find out if you are eligible. Reach out to the hospital before your medical service and explain your situation. If you do not qualify, the hospital may offer you a payment plan.
- Learn about your dental coverage options from local and state health programs, government insurance plans, dental schools, and dental clinical trials for people with limited incomes.
- You may qualify for financial assistance programs to help with eye exams, surgery, prescriptions, or glasses.

If you are uninsured or underinsured and must seek emergency medical treatment:

Under the Emergency Medical Treatment and Labor Act (EMTALA), you are guaranteed access to an emergency medical evaluation, even if you cannot pay. The act requires hospitals that receive Medicare funding and that provide emergency services to evaluate anyone who comes to their emergency room and requests treatment. If the evaluation confirms that you have an emergency medical condition, including active labor, they are then required to provide stabilizing treatment for you regardless of your ability to pay.

Section 23.2 | **Housing Resources for People with Disabilities**

This section includes text excerpted from "Financial Assistance and Support Services for People with Disabilities," USA.gov, December 12, 2019.

A variety of federal, state, and local housing programs can help you find and afford a place to live, modify an existing home for disabilities, or help you develop skills to live independently.

Each program has its own eligibility rules and application process.

RENTAL HOUSING

- People with disabilities are eligible for all public housing programs, rental assistance or subsidized housing, and Housing Choice (Section 8) voucher programs.
- You may also be eligible for a Non-Elderly Disabled (NED) Voucher, which helps people who are not seniors and have a disability get housing in a development traditionally set aside for seniors.
- Your state and your local city or county governments can explain any housing aid and programs for people with disabilities in your area.
- Certain Developments Vouchers can help nonelderly families that include a person with a disability find affordable rentals in housing developments limited to elderly residents.

HOMEOWNERSHIP

- If you are buying a home, Homeownership Vouchers can help pay mortgage and homeownership expenses.
- The U.S. Department of Agriculture (USDA) Rural Development program offers loans and grants for homeowners in rural areas for removing health hazards and making home modifications to accommodate a household member with a physical disability.

- If you are a veteran with a service-connected or age-related disability, you may be eligible for a housing grant to build or modify a home for your needs.

INDEPENDENT LIVING SKILLS

- State and local independent living centers can help you develop skills to live on your own with a disability.
- Contact your state to find out how its department of human services or disability office may be able to assist with modifications, housing counseling, locating rental housing, and independent living skills.

HOW DO I COMPLAIN?

You may require things such as ramps, grab bars, or service animals. It is illegal for housing providers to deny someone housing because of a disability or refuse to make reasonable accommodations for a tenant with a disability.

Section 23.3 | Getting Help Modifying My Vehicle for a Disability

This section includes text excerpted from "Financial Assistance and Support Services for People with Disabilities," USA.gov, December 12, 2019.

If you are thinking of adapting your vehicle for your disability, these tips on modifying or buying a vehicle can help.

GET FINANCIAL HELP BUYING A VEHICLE OR MODIFYING IT FOR DISABILITIES

Start by contacting your state vocational rehabilitation agency. The agency can point you to state grant and loan programs that may help cover costs. You can also look into other ways to pay. Depending on your situation and where you live, these can include:

- Local nonprofit organizations

- Your car insurance
- Workers' compensation
- Vehicle manufacturers
- Tax assistance

If you are a service member or veteran with a disability, you may qualify for help from the Department of Veterans Affairs (VA) to help pay for vehicle modifications.

FIND AND GET HELP PAYING FOR A DRIVER REHABILITATION SPECIALIST

A driver rehabilitation specialist (DRS) will identify the best vehicle modifications for you. They will give you advice on buying an adapted vehicle. To find a qualified DRS in your area, check with your local rehabilitation center.

Get Help Paying for an Evaluation

You may be able to find sources to cover part or the entire cost of your DRS evaluation.

Check with your:
- State vocational rehabilitation agency
- State workers' compensation official
- Health insurance company

Find a Qualified Mobility Dealer

Your DRS or rehabilitation agency can help you locate a qualified mobility equipment dealer to:
- Make sure you buy a vehicle that can be modified to meet your needs.
- Modify your vehicle.

GET TRAINING FOR YOUR VEHICLE'S NEW DISABILITY EQUIPMENT

If you are thinking of adapting your vehicle for your disability, these tips on modifying or buying a vehicle can help.

Section 23.4 | **Service Animals and Emotional Support Animals**

This section includes text excerpted from "Financial Assistance and Support Services for People with Disabilities," USA.gov, December 12, 2019.

Service animals are trained to complete work and tasks for the specific, individual needs of people with disabilities. Under the Americans with Disabilities Act (ADA), dogs may qualify as service animals. In some cases, the ADA also recognizes miniature horses as service animals. Emotional support animals serve as companions to people with disabilities but do not typically perform specific tasks or duties. They are not considered service animals under the ADA, but some state and local governments permit people to take them into public places.

If you are thinking about getting a service animal, first contact your medical provider. Find out if your disability is covered under the ADA and whether you need a service animal. Your doctor can help provide medical documentation and find a training program. You can also explore a list of service animal programs online, but make sure to research each organization's background and qualifications carefully.

WHAT DOES A SERVICE ANIMAL DO?
Common tasks include:
- Guiding a person who is blind
- Alerting someone who is deaf
- Aiding and protecting a person who is having a seizure
- Alerting a person with diabetes of high or low blood sugar
- Assisting someone in a wheelchair
- Calming a person with posttraumatic stress disorder (PTSD) during an anxiety attack

YOUR RIGHTS WITH SERVICE AND EMOTIONAL SUPPORT ANIMALS
- **General**. According to the ADA, state and local governments, businesses, and nonprofits that serve the

public must allow service animals to accompany people with disabilities where the public is typically allowed to go. Under certain state and local government laws, you may bring emotional support animals into public places.

- **Housing**. The Fair Housing Act (FHA) requires housing providers to permit or reasonably accommodate the use of service animals and emotional support animals by people with disabilities.
- **Travel**. The Air Carrier Access Act (ACAA) allows people with disabilities to travel with a service animal or emotional support animal.

LEARN ABOUT SERVICE AND EMOTIONAL SUPPORT ANIMALS FOR VETERANS

The VA provides guide dogs for blind or visually impaired veterans. It also offers service dogs for veterans with other disabilities. Benefits include veterinary care and equipment through VA Prosthetics and Sensory Aids.

The VA does not provide service dogs for veterans with mental disorders, such as PTSD. However, research is underway to see if dogs can help treat PTSD and its symptoms.

Section 23.5 | Achieving a Better Life Experience—Savings Accounts for People with Disabilities

This section includes text excerpted from "Financial Assistance and Support Services for People with Disabilities," USA.gov, December 12, 2019.

If you have a significant disability, you may be eligible to open a tax-free Achieving a Better Life Experience (ABLE) savings account. It can help you pay for education, housing, health, and other qualified disability expenses.

WHO IS ELIGIBLE FOR ABLE ACCOUNT?

- To be the designated beneficiary (owner) of the account, you must be blind or have a medical disability which occurred before 26 years of age.
- You may open only one ABLE account.
- You do not have to open an account in the state where you live. ABLE accounts are not currently available in every state. However, you can open one in any state with an active ABLE program.

CONTRIBUTING FUNDS TOWARD ABLE ACCOUNT

Find out who can contribute to or benefit from an ABLE account. Or, learn about how recently enacted tax laws and regulations apply to ABLE Savings accounts.

- The maximum annual contribution limit for your account is $15,000.
- You can exclude taxes on earnings and distributions (withdrawals) from the account. These deductions can help you pay for qualified disability expenses.

Keep in mind, the new tax law has made several changes to ABLE accounts:

- If you work, you can contribute your compensation toward your account along with the $15,000 limit. But, this additional contribution cannot be above the income poverty line for a one-person household.
- You may claim the Saver's Credit for your contributions to your ABLE account.
- Families can transfer or rollover funds from a 529 plan to an ABLE account. The account can benefit the account holder or another family member. This counts toward the $15,000 annual contribution limit.

MORE IMPORTANT ABLE ACCOUNT INFORMATION

The most important things to know about ABLE accounts, include:

- Where you can open an ABLE account

- Who can contribute to your account
- Examples of qualified disability expenses
- How other federal programs, such as Supplemental Security Income (SSI) and Medicaid, can affect your account.

Section 23.6 | Tax Help for People with Disabilities

This section includes text excerpted from "Financial Assistance and Support Services for People with Disabilities," USA.gov, December 12, 2019.

If you have a disability, you may be able to use Volunteer Income Tax Assistance (VITA) services to get free help with your taxes. The IRS also offers accessible tax forms and publications.

VOLUNTEER INCOME TAX ASSISTANCE

Volunteer Income Tax Assistance (VITA) offers free tax preparation help for people with disabilities. Find a VITA site near you.

Use the VITA/TCE checklist to learn more about the services of VITA and what you should bring to your appointment.

ACCESSIBLE TAX FORMS AND OTHER HELP

- Contact your local Internal Revenue Service (IRS) office for information on services for people with disabilities.
- Find tax forms and publications for people with disabilities at IRS.gov Accessibility. You will find a list of tax products to download that are accessible to a wide range of people. For hard copy braille or large print, call the IRS at 800-TAX-FORM (800-829-3676). Keep in mind, wait times may be long.
- Use the American Sign Language (ASL) videos created by the IRS.
- People with hearing impairments can contact the IRS by TTY/TDD 800-829-4059.

Section 23.7 | Organizations That Provide Help for People with Disabilities

This section includes text excerpted from "Financial Assistance and Support Services for People with Disabilities," USA.gov, December 12, 2019.

The following organizations provide services and information to people with disabilities:

- The National Council on Disability (NCD) is an independent federal agency that makes recommendations to the president and Congress to improve the quality of life (QOL) for Americans with disabilities and their families. The NCD works to empower individuals with disabilities and to promote equal opportunity.
- The National Disability Rights Network (NDRN) provides legally based advocacy services for people with disabilities in the United States.
- The U.S. Department of Education's Office of Special Education and Rehabilitative Services (OSERS) provides training and information for parents of children with disabilities and to people who work with them.
- The U.S. Department of Education (ED) has a list of State Special Education agencies to find educational resources and programs for people with disabilities.
- The U.S. Department of Housing and Urban Development's (HUD) Office of Fair Housing and Equal Opportunity (FHEO) offers resources and answers questions about the housing rights of people with disabilities, and the responsibilities of housing providers and building and design professionals according to the federal law.
- The National Library Service for the Blind and Physically Handicapped (NLS) administers a free loan service of recorded and braille books and magazines, music scores in braille and large print, plus specially

designed playback equipment. Service is also extended to eligible American citizens residing abroad. While NLS administers the program, direct service is provided through a national network of cooperating libraries.

- The National Center on Health, Physical Activity and Disability (NCHPAD) is a resource center that works to help people with disabilities get healthier by participating more in all types of physical and social activities. The NCHPAD also trains service providers to make their programs more inclusive.
- Special Olympics is a global organization that changes lives by promoting understanding, acceptance, and inclusion among people with and without intellectual disabilities through year-round sports, health, education, and community building held around the world.
- American Foundation for the Blind (AFB) removes barriers, creates solutions, and expands possibilities so people with vision loss can achieve their full potential.

TELECOMMUNICATIONS RELAY SERVICES

Telecommunications relay services for people with hearing or speaking disabilities—link telephone conversations between individuals who use standard voice telephones and those who use the text telephones (TTYs). Calls can be made from either type of telephone to the other type through the relay service.

Local Relay Services

States provide relay services for local and long-distance calls. Consult your local telephone directory or list from the Federal Communications Commission (FCC) for information on the use, fees (if any), services, and dialing instructions for your area.

Federal Relay Service

The Federal Relay Service (FRS) is a program of the U.S. General Services Administration (GSA). It provides access to TTY users to conduct official business nationwide with and within the federal government. The toll-free number is 800-377-8642. For more information on relay communications or to obtain a brochure on using the FRS, please call toll-free 800-877-0996.

Other Telephone Services

If you use a TTY, you can receive operator and directory assistance for calls by calling toll-free 800-855-1155.

Part 5 | **Reducing the Risk of Traumatic Brain Injury**

Chapter 24 | **Preventing Traumatic Brain Injury**

Traumatic brain injury (TBI) is a disruption in the normal function of the brain that can be caused by a bump, blow, or jolt to the head, or penetrating head injury. There are many ways to reduce the chances of sustaining a traumatic brain injury.

You can prevent traumatic brain injury by doing the following:
- Buckle up every ride—Wear a seat belt every time you drive—or ride—in a motor vehicle.
- Never drive while under the influence of alcohol or drugs.
- Wear a helmet, or appropriate headgear, when you or your children:
    - Ride a bike, motorcycle, snowmobile, scooter, or use an all-terrain vehicle
    - Play a contact sport such as football, ice hockey, or boxing
    - Use in-line skates or ride a skateboard
    - Bat and run bases in baseball or softball
    - Ride a horse
    - Ski or snowboard
- Prevent older adult falls.
    - Talk to your doctor to evaluate your risk for falling, and talk with them about specific things you can do to reduce your risk for a fall.

This chapter contains text excerpted from the following sources: Text in this chapter begins with excerpts from "Traumatic Brain Injury and Concussion," Centers for Disease Control and Prevention (CDC), March 4, 2019; Text under the heading "Funded Programs, Activities, and Research" is excerpted from "Traumatic Brain Injury Prevention," Centers for Disease Control and Prevention (CDC), January 14, 2020.

- Ask your doctor or pharmacist to review your medicines to see if any of them might make you dizzy or sleepy. This should include prescription medicines, over-the-counter (OTC) medicines, herbal supplements, and vitamins.
- Have your eyes checked at least once a year, and be sure to update your eyeglasses if needed.
- Do strength and balance exercises to make your legs stronger and improve your balance.
- Make your home safer.
- Make living and play areas safer for children.
  - Install window guards to keep young children from falling out of open windows.
  - Use safety gates at the top and bottom of stairs when young children are around.
  - Make sure your child's playground has soft material under it, such as hardwood mulch or sand.

FUNDED PROGRAMS, ACTIVITIES, AND RESEARCH

Traumatic brain injuries contribute to about 30 percent of all injury deaths. Every day, 153 people in the United States die from injuries that include a TBI. People who survive a TBI can face effects that last a few days, or the rest of their lives. TBIs can cause impaired thinking or memory, movement, sensation (such as vision or hearing), or emotional functioning (such as personality changes or depression). These issues not only affect individuals but can have lasting effects on families and communities.

The Centers for Disease Control and Prevention (CDC) research and programs work to prevent TBIs and help people recognize, respond, and recover if a TBI occurs. Eight International Committee of the Red Cross (ICRC) is working to address TBI through research, training, or outreach activities:
- Columbia University
- Icahn School of Medicine at Mount Sinai (ISMMS)
- Johns Hopkins School of Public Health (JHSPH)
- The Research Institute at Nationwide Children's Hospital

- University of Iowa
- University of Michigan
- University of North Carolina at Chapel Hill
- University of Pennsylvania

Research: Studying Ways to Prevent Traumatic Brain Injury

Examples of the CDC-funded ICRC research projects are listed here:

- Exploring Universal Bicycle Helmet Policies: A Translation Research Study (JHSPH)
- Head Impact Biomechanics as a Behavior Modification Tool to Reduce Mild Traumatic Brain Injury Risk (University of North Carolina at Chapel Hill)
- Impact of Ohio's Youth Concussion Law on Patterns of Healthcare Utilization (The Research Institute at Nationwide Children's Hospital)
- The Juvenile Justice System and Traumatic Brain Injury (ISMMS)

Outreach: Putting Research into Action to Prevent Traumatic Brain Injury

The Mount Sinai Injury Control Research Center (MS-ICRC) used a research method called "verbal autopsy" to gather health information about TBI patients who survive their injuries but then subsequently die. Verbal autopsy involves talking to the patient's family about the patient's health in the year before the patient died. MS-ICRC worked with the TBI Model System Centers to implement the verbal autopsy research method when TBI patients later die. Since implementation, the Centers' clinicians and researchers better understand the importance of monitoring post-TBI health and helping to learn more about post-TBI health challenges by tracking the health of TBI patients in their first year after injury.

The Johns Hopkins Center for Injury Research and Policy (CIRP) developed a 4-minute video about bicycle helmet safety to directly reach urban, minority youth. This You Make the Call video was part of a larger pilot program that also provided a free helmet, a helmet fitting, and safety instructions by a health educator. The pilot included 20 pairs of parents and children. Children who participated were about 10 years of age and included equal numbers of boys and girls. The majority of these children reported daily or weekly bike-riding (65%). None of the 20 children reported that they "always" wore a helmet while bike-riding. 16 of the children (80%) reported that they "never" wore a helmet. 16 of the children (80%) did not own a helmet. A month after the intervention, youth who reported bike-riding also reported significantly higher helmet use. The follow-up visit included 12 of the children. Five children reported that they "always" use their helmets, compared to 0 before the intervention. There was also an increase from 35 to 66 percent in youth reporting that parents required helmet use. The project received a Gold Winner and Best in Show awards from the National Health Information Awards program. CIRP is sharing this important work through national and international conference presentations and academic papers.

Since 2012, the Penn Injury Science Center at the University of Pennsylvania has collaborated with multiple institutions in the Big Ten and Ivy League sports conferences to collect concussion data on varsity athletes in a surveillance system. The study collects information in real-time from students playing all types of sports. Each athlete is monitored to determine how long it takes for symptoms to resolve and how long it takes to return to academic and physical activities. Since 2012, more than 2,000 concussion cases have been entered into the surveillance system. In 2017, the Penn Injury Science Center (PISC) ICRC partnered with the Big Ten—Ivy League Traumatic Brain Injury Research Collaboration to take over operations of the surveillance system and to conduct analyses for the study. The Research Collaboration's work is already showing the difference interventions can make. The Ivy League conference averaged six concussions per season during kickoff plays from 2012 to 2015. In 2016, new kickoff return rules were put in place, and athletes suffered zero concussions on kickoff plays that year.

Training: Building the Field to Prevent Traumatic Brain Injury

The University of Iowa Injury Prevention Research Center (UI IPRC) developed an inventory of evidence-based bicycle safety programs. Bicycling for children comes with benefits but there are risks to consider. Education is an important piece to increasing child bicycle safety. There are numerous child bicycle education programs throughout the United States but no single program is recognized as the best intervention. Educators can use this inventory to identify critical components or how to improve programs in their area. Common program elements are grouped by age. This inventory provides a foundation that child bicycle education standards can be built upon.

The Mount Sinai Injury Control Research Center (MS-ICRC) developed the Executive Plus and Short-Term Executive Plus (STEP) programs that help TBI patients deal with challenges in solving problems and controlling their emotions after their injuries, and a free manual to help other organizations implement these programs. MS-ICRC's assessment of the program implementation showed that the programs were not working as well as expected. However, MS-ICRC identified three sites that had successfully used the Smart Traveler Enrollment Program (STEP) and investigated why the program had worked in those facilities. MS-ICRC is now sharing what it learned to improve the implementation of the STEP program and the manual more widespread and successful.

The University of Michigan Injury Prevention Center (UMIPC) developed a massive open online course (MOOC) focusing on a number of injury-related public-health areas, including epidemiology, surveillance, risk and protective factors, suicide prevention, and sports injury prevention. The MOOC includes 59 video learning segments grouped into themes and taught by a panel of 25 nationally recognized injury prevention experts. Learners can gain new skills to improve clinical practice, support families and their communities, and learn detailed strategies and techniques to apply best injury prevention practices. One of the MOOC's modules focuses on concussion prevention. In this module, learners can learn what concussions are, how often people get them, how they are diagnosed and treated, and the long-term effects of concussions. In the first four months after launch, more than 1500 learners enrolled and expanded the University of Michigan's reach to rural populations.

Chapter 25 | **Preventing Falls in Elderly**

SPEAK UP

Talk openly with your loved one and their healthcare provider about fall risks and prevention.

- Tell a healthcare provider right away if your loved one has fallen, or if they are worried about falling, or seem unsteady.
- Keep an updated list of your loved one's medications. Show a healthcare provider or pharmacist all of their medications, including over-the-counter (OTC) medications, and supplements. Discuss any side effects, like feeling dizzy or sleepy
- Ask their healthcare provider about taking vitamin D supplements to improve bone, muscle, and nerve health.

KEEP MOVING

Activities that improve balance and strengthen legs (like Tai Chi) can prevent falls.

- Exercise and movement can also help your loved one feel better and more confident.

This chapter contains text excerpted from the following sources: Text beginning with the heading "Speak Up" is excerpted from "Family Caregivers: Protect Your Loved Ones from Falling," Centers for Disease Control and Prevention (CDC), 2018; Text under the heading "Home Fall Prevention Checklist" is excerpted from "Check for Safety a Home Fall Prevention Checklist for Older Adults," Centers for Disease Control and Prevention (CDC), 2017.

- Check with their healthcare provider about the best type of exercise program for them.

HAVE EYES AND FEET CHECKED
Being able to see and walk comfortably can prevent falls.
- Have their eyes checked by an eye doctor at least once a year
- Replace eyeglasses as needed.
- Have their healthcare provider check their feet once a year.
- Discuss proper footwear, and ask whether seeing a foot specialist is advised.

MAKE THE HOME SAFE
Most falls happen at home.
- Keep floors clutter-free.
- Remove small throw rugs, or use double-sided tape to keep the rugs from slipping.
- Add grab bars in the bathroom—next to and inside the tub, and next to the toilet.
- Have handrails and lights installed on all staircases
- Make sure the home has lots of light.

HOME FALL PREVENTION CHECKLIST
Stairs and Steps (Indoors and Outdoors)
- Always keep objects off the stairs.
- Fix loose or uneven steps.
- Have an electrician put in an overhead light and light switch at the top and bottom of the stairs. You can get light switches that glow.
- Have a friend or family member change the light bulb.
- Make sure the carpet is firmly attached to every step, or remove the carpet and attach nonslip rubber treads to the stairs.
- Fix loose handrails, or put in new ones. Make sure handrails are on both sides of the stairs, and are as long as the stairs.

Floors

- Ask someone to move the furniture so your path is clear.
- Remove the rugs, or use double-sided tape or a nonslip backing so the rugs will not slip.
- Pick up things that are on the floor. Always keep objects off the floor.
- Coil or tape cords and wires next to the wall so you cannot trip over them. If needed, have an electrician put in another outlet.

Kitchen

- Keep things you use often on the lower shelves (about waist high).
- If you must use a step stool, get one with a bar to hold on to. Never use a chair as a step stool.

Bedrooms

- Place a lamp close to the bed where it is easy to reach.
- Put in a nightlight so you can see where you are walking. Some nightlights go on by themselves after dark.

Bathrooms

- Put a nonslip rubber mat or self-stick strips on the floor of the tub or shower.
- Have grab bars put in next to and inside the tub, and next to the toilet.

Chapter 26 | Stay Safe on Roads

Chapter Contents

Section 26.1 | **Drive Safe on the Roads**

This section contains text excerpted from the following sources: Text under the heading "Summer Driving Tips" is excerpted from "Summer Driving Tips 2019," National Highway Traffic Safety Administration (NHTSA), 2019; Text under the heading "Winter Driving Tips" is excerpted from "Winter Driving Tips," National Highway Traffic Safety Administration (NHTSA), February 22, 2017.

SUMMER DRIVING TIPS

Of the many great things about summertime, few match the fun of a family road trip. Before you hook up that new boat or camper, or hit the road with your family or friends in your car, sport utility vehicle (SUV), pickup, or recreational vehicle (RV), take the time to review these summer travel safety tips. Prevention and planning may take a little time up-front, but will spare you from dealing with the consequences of a breakdown—or worse yet, a highway crash—later.

Before You Go
GET YOUR CAR SERVICED

Regular maintenance such as tune-ups, oil changes, battery checks, and tire rotations go a long way toward preventing breakdowns. If your vehicle has been serviced according to the manufacturer's recommendations, it should be in good condition to travel. If not—or you do not know the service history of the vehicle you plan to drive—schedule a preventive maintenance checkup with your mechanic right away.

CHECK FOR RECALLS

Owners may not always know that their vehicle has been recalled and needs to be repaired. The National Highway Traffic Safety Administration (NHTSA), Vehicle Identification Number (VIN) look-up tool lets you enter a VIN to quickly learn if a specific vehicle has not been repaired as part of a safety recall in the last 15 years. Check for recalls on your vehicle by searching now on NHTSA.gov/Recalls and sign up for email recall alerts at NHTSA.gov/Alerts.

GO OVER YOUR VEHICLE SAFETY CHECKLIST

Regardless of how well you take care of your ride, it is important to perform the following basic safety checks before you go on a road trip:

Tires

Air pressure, tread wear, spare. Check your vehicle's tire inflation pressure at least once a month and when your tires are cold (when the car has not been driven for three hours or more)—and do not forget to check your spare, if your vehicle is equipped with one. The correct pressure for your tires is listed on a label on the driver's door pillar or doorframe or in the vehicle owner's manual—the correct pressure for your vehicle is not the number listed on the tire itself. A tire does not have to be punctured to lose air. All tires naturally lose some air over time and become underinflated. In fact, underinflation is the leading cause of tire failure.

Also, take 5 minutes to inspect your tires for signs of excessive or uneven wear. If the tread is worn down to 2/32 of an inch, it is time to replace your tires. Look for the built-in wear bar indicators on your tires or use the "penny test" to determine when it is time to replace your tires. Place a penny in the tread with Lincoln's head upside down. If you can see the top of Lincoln's head, your vehicle needs new tires. If you find uneven wear across the tires' tread, it means your tires need rotation and/or your wheels need to be aligned before you travel.

Lights

Headlights, brake lights, turn signals, emergency flashers, interior lights, and trailer lights. See and be seen! Make sure all the lights on your vehicle are in working order. Check your headlights, brake lights, turn signals, emergency flashers, and interior lights. Towing a trailer? Be sure to also check your trailer including brake lights and turn signals. A failure of the trailer light connection is a common problem and a serious safety hazard.

Cooling System

Coolant level and servicing. The radiator in your vehicle needs water and antifreeze (coolant) to keep your engine functioning properly. When your car has not been running and the engine is completely cool, carefully check your coolant level to make sure the reservoir is full. In addition, if your coolant is clear, looks rusty, or has particles floating in it, it is time to have your cooling system flushed and refilled. If your coolant looks sludgy or oily, immediately take your vehicle to a mechanic.

Fluid Level

Oil, brake, transmission, power steering, and windshield washer fluids. Check your vehicle's oil level periodically. As with coolant, if it is time or even nearly time to have the oil changed, now would be a good time to do it. In addition, check the following fluid levels: brake, automatic transmission or clutch, power steering, and windshield washer. Make sure each reservoir is full; if you see any signs of fluid leakage, take your vehicle in to be serviced.

Belts and Hoses

Condition and fittings. Look under the hood and inspect all belts and hoses to make sure there are no signs of bulges, blisters, cracks, or cuts in the rubber. High summer temperatures accelerate the rate at which rubber belts and hoses degrade, so it is best to replace them now if they show signs of obvious wear. While you are at it, check all hose connections to make sure they are secure.

Wiper Blades

Wear and tear on both sides. After the heavy toll imposed by winter storms and spring rains, windshield wiper blades may need to be replaced. Like rubber belts and hoses, wiper blades are vulnerable to the summer heat. Examine your blades for signs of wear and tear on both sides. The blades can also deform and fail to work properly in both directions. If they are not in top condition, invest in new ones before you go.

Air Conditioning

A/C check. Check A/C performance before traveling. Lack of air conditioning on a hot summer day affects people who are in poor health or who are sensitive to heat, such as children and older adults.

Floor Mats

Proper size and correct installation. Improperly installed floor mats in your vehicle may interfere with the operation of the accelerator or brake pedal, increasing the risk of a crash.

- Remove old floor mats before the installation of new mats; never stack mats.
- Use mats that are the correct size and fit for your vehicle.
- Follow the manufacturer's instructions for mat installation. Use available retention clips to secure the mat and prevent it from sliding forward.
- Every time the mats are removed for any reason, verify that the driver's mat is reinstalled correctly.

PACK AN EMERGENCY ROADSIDE KIT

Even a well-maintained vehicle can break down, so it is advisable to put together an emergency roadside kit to carry with you. A cell phone tops the list of suggested emergency kit contents since it allows you to call for help when and while you need it. Suggested emergency roadside kit contents:

- Cell phone and charger
- First-aid kit
- Flashlight
- Flares and a white flag
- Jumper cables
- Tire pressure gauge
- Jack (and ground mat) for changing a tire
- Work gloves and a change of clothes
- Basic repair tools and some duct tape (for temporarily repairing a hose leak)
- Water and paper towels for cleaning up
- Nonperishable food, drinking water, and medicines
- Extra windshield washer fluid

- Maps
- Emergency blankets, towels, and coats

Safety First
PROTECT YOURSELF AND YOUR LOVED ONES
Buckle up—every trip—every time. All passengers must agree to wear their seat belts every time they are riding in your vehicle. Set the example by always wearing your seat belt.

PROTECT THE CHILDREN
When traveling with children, take every precaution to keep them safe.
- All children under 13 years of age should ride in the back seat.
- Make sure car seats and booster seats are properly installed and that any children riding with you are in the correct car seat, booster seat, or wear seat belt that is appropriate for their size. All passengers in your vehicle should be buckled up on every trip, every time.
- Click on the NHTSA's child passenger safety recommendations to find out how to select the right seat for your child's age and size.
- Never leave your child unattended in or around a vehicle.
- Always remember to lock your vehicle when exiting so children do not play or get trapped inside.

On the Road
STAY ALERT
Remember that long trips can be tough on children—and, in turn, tough on you. Plan enough time to stop along the way to take a group stretch, get something to eat and drink, return any calls or text messages, and change drivers if you are feeling tired or drowsy. Consider staying overnight at a hotel or family resort. It can make the trip easier and less tiring for everyone—and more of

an adventure, too. Bring along a few favorite books, videos, or soft toys to keep little ones content and occupied. The trip will seem to go faster for them, and keep you from being distracted every time they ask, "Are we there yet?"

Long-distance driving can be tedious, and it is tempting to look for something to distract you to make the time pass faster. But when you are the driver, your only responsibility is to keep your eyes on the road, hands on the wheel, and concentration on the task of driving. No loss of life–neither your passengers nor any other road users–are worth a phone call or text. And remember, law enforcement officers across the nation are now using innovative strategies to aggressively enforce their state distracted driving laws.

SHARE THE ROAD

Warmer weather attracts many types of roadway users, including motorcyclists, bicyclists, and pedestrians.

While they have the same rights, privileges, and responsibilities as every motorist, these road users are more vulnerable because they do not have the protection of a car or truck.

Leave more distance between you and a motorcycle—three or four seconds worth. Motorcycles are much lighter than other vehicles and can stop in much shorter distances.

Always signal your intentions before changing lanes or merging with traffic. This allows other road users to anticipate your movement and find a safe lane position.

Be mindful of pedestrians. Things to remember as a driver:

- You can encounter pedestrians anytime and anywhere.
- Distracted walking is becoming part of the distracted traffic epidemic. Keep your eyes open for distracted pedestrians.
- Pedestrians can be very hard to see—especially in bad weather or at night.
- Stop for pedestrians who are in a crosswalk, even if it is not marked. This will help drivers in the other lanes see the pedestrians in time to stop.
- Cars stopped in the street may be stopped to allow pedestrians to cross. Do not pass if there is any doubt.

- Do not assume that pedestrians can see you or that they will act predictably. They may be distracted, or physically or mentally impaired.
- When you are turning and waiting for a gap in traffic, watch for pedestrians who may have moved into your intended path.
- Be especially attentive around schools and in neighborhoods where children are active. Drive the way you want people to drive in front of your own home.

AVOID RISKY DRIVING BEHAVIORS
Distracted Driving

The focus of every driver, at all times, should be driving.

Distracted driving is anything that takes your attention away from driving. The most obvious forms of distraction are cell phone use, texting while driving, eating, drinking, talking with passengers, and using in-vehicle technologies and portable electronic devices.

Set down some safety rules with your co-drivers before you hit the road. These rules should include refraining from activities that take your eyes and attention off the road. Insist that your co-drivers agree to make every effort to move to a safe place off of the road before using a cell phone—even in an emergency.

Impaired Driving

Alcohol and drugs can impair perception, judgment, motor skills, and memory—the skills critical for safe and responsible driving. Deaths caused by impaired driving are preventable, and too many lives are tragically cut short in traffic crashes involving alcohol- and drug-impaired driving. Impaired driving not only puts the driver at risk—it threatens the lives of passengers and all others who share the road. Every year it causes the deaths of thousands of loved ones. Be responsible; do not drink and drive. Illegal drugs, as well as prescription and over-the-counter (OTC) medications, can be just as deadly on the road as alcohol. If you plan to drink, designate a sober driver before going out.

Speeding

Obey all posted speed limits, or drive slower if necessary based on weather or traffic conditions.

Summer Safety
KEEP KIDS SAFE IN AND AROUND THE CAR

There are other dangers to children in and around cars that you should know. One of those dangers is hyperthermia, or heatstroke. Heatstroke can occur when a child is left unattended in a parked vehicle or gains unsupervised access. Never leave children alone in the car—not even for a few minutes or with the engine running. Vehicles heat up quickly; if the outside temperature is in the low 80s, the temperature inside the vehicle can reach deadly levels in just a few minutes—even with a window rolled down. A child's body temperature rises three to five times faster than that of an adult.

Before you back out of a driveway or parking spot, prevent backovers by walking around your vehicle to check for children running and playing. When using a backup camera, remember that kids, pets, and objects may still be out of view but in the path of your vehicle. When children play, they are often oblivious to cars and trucks around them. They may believe that motorists will watch out for them. Furthermore, every vehicle has a blind zone. As the size and height of a vehicle increases, so does the blind zone area. Large vehicles, trucks, SUVs, RVs, and vans, are more likely than cars to be involved in backovers.

Be sure to lock your vehicle's doors at all times when it is not in use. Put the keys somewhere that children cannot get to them. Children who enter vehicles on their own with no adult supervision can be killed or injured by power windows, seat belt entanglement, vehicle rollaway, heatstroke, or trunk entrapment.

WINTER DRIVING TIPS
Before You Go
GET YOUR CAR SERVICED

Visit your mechanic for a tune-up and ask them to check for leaks, badly worn hoses or other needed parts, repairs, and replacements.

CHECK FOR RECALLS

The NHTSA's Recalls Look-up Tool lets you enter a vehicle identification number (VIN) to quickly learn if your vehicle has a critical safety issue that has not been repaired, and how to get that repair done for free.

KNOW YOUR CAR

Read your vehicle's manual to familiarize yourself with the features on your vehicle—such as antilock brakes and electronic stability control—and how the features perform in wintry conditions. When renting a car, become familiar with the vehicle before driving it off the lot.

PLUG IT IN

For electric and hybrid-electric vehicles, minimize the drain on the battery. If the vehicle has a thermal heating pack for the battery, plug your vehicle in whenever it is not in use. Preheat the passenger compartment before you unplug your vehicle in the morning.

STOCK YOUR VEHICLE

Carry items in your vehicle to handle common winter driving-related tasks or supplies you might need in an emergency, including the following:
- Snow shovel, broom, and ice scraper
- Abrasive material, such as sand or kitty litter, in case your vehicle gets stuck in the snow
- Jumper cables, flashlight, and warning devices, such as flares and emergency markers
- Blankets for protection from the cold
- A cell phone with charger, water, food, and any necessary medicine (for longer trips or when driving in lightly populated areas)

PLAN YOUR TRAVEL AND ROUTE

Before heading out, make sure to check the weather, road conditions, and traffic. Do not rush through your trip, and allow plenty of time to get to your destination safely. And always familiarize yourself with directions and maps before you go, even if you use a Global Positioning System (GPS), and let others know your route and anticipated arrival time.

GO OVER YOUR VEHICLE SAFETY CHECKLIST
Battery
When the temperature drops, so does battery power. For gasoline and diesel engines, it takes more battery power to start your vehicle in cold weather. For electric and hybrid-electric vehicles, the driving range is reduced when the battery is cold. Have your mechanic check your battery, charging system, and belts, and have them make any necessary repairs or replacements. For hybrid-electric vehicles, keep gasoline in the tank to support the gasoline engine.

Lights
Check your headlights, brake lights, turn signals, emergency flashers, and interior lights. Be sure to also check your trailer brake lights and turn signals, if necessary.

Cooling System
Make sure you have enough coolant in your vehicle, and that the coolant meets the manufacturer's specifications. See your vehicle owner's manual for specific recommendations on coolant. You or a mechanic should check the cooling system for leaks, test the coolant, and drain or replace old coolant as needed.

Windshield Wipers
Washer Reservoir. You can go through a lot of windshield wiper fluid fairly quickly in a single snowstorm, so be prepared for whatever might come your way by ensuring your vehicle's reservoir is full of high-quality winter fluid with de-icer before winter weather hits.

Wipers and Defrosters. Make sure defrosters and windshield wipers—both front and rear work, and replace any worn blades.

You may also want to consider installing heavy-duty winter wipers if you live in an area that gets a lot of snow and ice.

Floor Mats

Improperly installed floor mats in your vehicle may interfere with the operation of the accelerator or brake pedal, increasing the risk of a crash. Be sure to follow the manufacturer's instructions for mat installation, use retention clips to secure the mat and prevent it from sliding forward, and always use mats that are the correct size and fit for your vehicle.

Tires

As the outside temperature drops, so does tire inflation pressure. Make sure each tire is filled to the vehicle manufacturer's recommended inflation pressure, which is listed in your owner's manual and on a placard located on the driver's side door frame. The correct pressure is NOT the number listed on the tire. Be sure to check tires when they are cold, which means the car has not been driven for at least three hours. Read through for safe tire tips:

- Regardless of season, inspect your tires at least once a month and before long road trips. It only takes about five minutes. If you find yourself driving under less-than-optimal road conditions this winter, you will be glad you took the time. Do not forget to check your spare tire.
- If you plan to use snow tires, have them installed in the fall so you are prepared before it snows. Check out www.nhtsa.gov/tires for tire ratings before buying new ones, and look for winter tires with the snowflake symbol.
- Look closely at your tread and replace tires that have uneven wear or insufficient tread. Tread should be at least 2/32 of an inch or greater on all tires.
- Check the age of each tire. Some vehicle manufacturers recommend that tires be replaced every six years regardless of use, but check your owner's manual to find out.

Safety First
PROTECT YOURSELF AND YOUR LOVED ONES

Always wear your seat belt every trip, every time—and ensure that everyone else in your vehicle is buckled-up in age- and size-appropriate car seats, booster seats, or seat belts.

PROTECT YOUR CHILDREN

- Remember that all children under 13 years of age should always ride properly buckled in the back seat.
- Make sure car seats and booster seats are properly installed and that any children riding with you are in the right seat for their ages and sizes. See the NHTSA's child passenger safety recommendations to find out how to select the right car seat for your child's age and size.
- Though thick outerwear will keep your children warm, it can interfere with the proper harness fit on your child in a car seat. Choose thin, warm layers for your child instead, and place blankets or coats around your child after the harness is snug and secure for extra warmth.
- Never leave your child unattended in or around your vehicle.
- Always remember to lock your vehicle and to keep your keys out of reach when exiting so children do not play or get trapped inside.

On the Road
STAY ALERT

Keep your gas tank close to full whenever possible, and, on longer trips, plan enough time to stop to stretch, get something to eat, return calls or text messages, and change drivers or rest if you feel drowsy.

AVOID RISKY DRIVING BEHAVIORS

You know the rules: Do not text or drive distracted; obey posted speed limits; and always drive sober. Both alcohol and drugs whether legal or illicit can cause impairment. It is illegal to drive impaired by any substance in all states—no exceptions. Alcohol and drugs can impair the skills critical for safe and responsible driving such as coordination, judgment, perception, and reaction time.

DRIVING IN WINTER CONDITIONS

Slow down. It is harder to control or stop your vehicle on a slick or snow-covered surface.

NAVIGATING AROUND SNOW PLOWS

Do not crowd a snow plow or travel beside it. Snow plows travel slowly, make wide turns, stop often, overlap lanes, and exit the road frequently. However, the road behind an active snow plow is safer to drive on. If you find yourself behind a snow plow, stay behind it or use caution when passing.

In an Emergency
WHAT TO DO IN A WINTER EMERGENCY

If you are stopped or stalled in wintry weather, follow these safety rules:

- Stay with your car and do not overexert yourself.
- Put bright markers on the antenna or windows and keep the interior dome light turned on.
- To avoid asphyxiation from carbon monoxide poisoning, do not run your car for long periods of time with the windows up or in an enclosed space. If you must run your vehicle, clear the exhaust pipe of any snow and run it only sporadically—just long enough to stay warm.

Section 26.2 | **Wear Seat Belts**

This section includes text excerpted from "Seat Belts: Get the Facts," Centers for Disease Control and Prevention (CDC), June 5, 2018.

THE PROBLEM
How Big Is the Problem of Crash-Related Injuries and Deaths to Drivers and Passengers?

Motor vehicle crashes are a leading cause of death among those 1 to 54 years of age in the United States. Most crash-related deaths in the United States occur in drivers and passengers.

For adults and older children (who are big enough for seat belts to fit properly), seat belt use is one of the most effective ways to save lives and reduce injuries in crashes. Yet millions do not buckle up on every trip.

DEATHS

- A total of 23,714 drivers and passengers in passenger vehicles died in motor vehicle crashes in 2016.
- More than half (range: 53 to 62%) of teens (13 to 19 years of age) and adults 20 to 44 years of age who died in crashes in 2016 were not buckled up at the time of the crash.

INJURIES

- More than 2.6 million drivers and passengers were treated in emergency departments (ED) as a result of being injured in motor vehicle crashes in 2016.
- Young adult drivers and passengers (18 to 24 years of age) have the highest crash-related nonfatal injury rates of all adults.

COSTS

- Nonfatal crash injuries to drivers and passengers resulted in more than $48 billion in lifetime medical and work loss costs in 2010.

RISK FACTORS
Who Is Least Likely to Wear a Seat Belt?
AGE

- Young adults (18 to 24 years of age) are less likely to wear seat belts than those in older age groups.

GENDER

- Men are less likely to wear seat belts than women.

METROPOLITAN STATUS

- Adults who live in nonmetropolitan areas are less likely to wear seat belts than adults who live in metropolitan areas.

STATE LAWS

- Seat belt use is lower in states with secondary enforcement seat belt laws or no seat belt laws (86% in 2017) compared to states with primary enforcement laws (91% in 2017).

Seating Position in Vehicle

- Rear-seat motor vehicle passengers are less likely than front-seat passengers to wear a seat belt, making them more likely to injure themselves and drivers or other passengers in a crash.

EFFECTIVENESS
What Is the Impact of Seat Belt Use?

- Seat belts reduce serious crash-related injuries and deaths by about half.
- Seat belts saved almost 15,000 lives in 2016.
- Airbags provide added protection but are not a substitute for seat belts. Airbags plus seat belts provide the greatest protection for adults.

Primary Enforcement Laws Make a Difference

Research shows primary enforcement seat belt laws make a big difference in getting more people to buckle up. Observed seat belt use in 2017 was 91 percent in states with primary enforcement laws but only 86 percent in states with secondary enforcement laws or no seat belt laws.

A primary enforcement seat belt law means a police officer can pull a vehicle over and issue a ticket just because a driver or passenger covered by the law is not wearing a seat belt. A secondary enforcement law only allows a police officer to issue a ticket for someone not wearing a seat belt if the driver has been pulled over for some other offense. State primary and secondary seat belt laws vary by whether driver and front seat passengers are required to be buckled or whether drivers and all passengers (i.e., front and rear seats) are required to be buckled. These requirements may also vary depending on the age of the passenger.

PREVENTION
What Can Be Done to Increase Seat Belt Use among Adults?

When it comes to increasing seat belt use, individuals, government, and health professionals can help promote safety.

States can:

- Consider proven strategies for increasing seat belt use and reducing child motor vehicle injuries and deaths, which include:
  - Primary enforcement seat belt laws, which have been shown to increase use and reduce deaths compared with secondary enforcement laws
  - Seat belt laws that apply to everyone in the car, not just those in the front seat
  - Fines for not wearing a seatbelt that are high enough to be effective
- Make sure that police and state troopers enforce all seat belt laws.
- Support seat belt laws with visible police presence and awareness campaigns for the public.
- Educate the public to make seatbelt use a social norm.

Health professionals can:
- Remind patients about the importance of seat belt use.
- Encourage patients to make wearing seatbelt a habit.
- Wear seat belts themselves and encourage their colleagues to do the same

Parents and caregivers can:
- Use a seat belt on every trip, no matter how short. This sets a good example.
- Make sure children are properly buckled up in a car seat, booster seat, or seat belt, whichever is appropriate for their age, height, and weight.
- Have all children 12 years of age and under sit properly buckled in the back seat.
- Remember to never place a rear-facing child safety seat in front of an airbag.
- Properly buckle children in the middle back seat when possible because it is the safest spot in the vehicle.

Everyone can:
- Use a seat belt on every trip, no matter how short.
- Require everyone in the car to buckle up, including those in the back seat.

Section 26.3 | **Motorcycle Safety**

This section contains text excerpted from the following sources: Text in this section begins with excerpts from "Motorcycle Safety," National Highway Traffic Safety Administration (NHTSA), February 22, 2005. Reviewed May 2020; Text under the heading "Choose the Right Motorcycle Helmet" is excerpted from "Choose the Right Motorcycle Helmet," National Highway Traffic Safety Administration (NHTSA), May 17, 2019.

The number of motorcyclists killed in crashes dropped to 4,985 in 2018, an almost 5 percent decrease, but motorcycle riders are still overrepresented in traffic fatalities. To keep everyone safe, the National Highway Traffic Safety Administration (NHTSA) urges drivers and motorcyclists to share the road and be alert, and also reminds motorcyclists to make themselves visible, to use DOT-compliant motorcycle helmets, and to always ride sober.

MOTORIST AWARENESS

Safe riding practices and cooperation from all road users will help reduce the number of fatalities and injuries on our nation's highways. But, it is especially important for drivers to understand the safety challenges faced by motorcyclists, such as size and visibility, and motorcycle riding practices like downshifting and weaving to know how to anticipate and respond to them. By raising motorists' awareness, both drivers and riders will be safer sharing the road.

MOTORCYCLIST SAFETY

If you ride a motorcycle, you already know how much fun riding can be. You understand the exhilaration of cruising the open road and the challenge of controlling a motorcycle. But, motorcycling also can be dangerous. The latest data on vehicle miles traveled shows that motorcyclists are about 28 times as likely as passenger car occupants to die in a motor vehicle traffic crash. Safe motorcycling takes balance, coordination, and good judgment.

ROAD READY
Make Sure You Are Properly Licensed

Driving a car and riding a motorcycle require different skills and knowledge. Although motorcycle-licensing regulations vary, all states require a motorcycle license endorsement to supplement your automobile driver's license. To receive the proper endorsement in most states, you will need to pass written and on-cycle skills tests administered by your state's licensing agency. Some states require you to take a state-sponsored rider education course. Others waive the on-cycle skills test if you have already taken and passed a state-approved course. Either way, completing a motorcycle rider education course is a good way to ensure you have the correct instruction and experience it takes to ride a motorcycle.

Contact your state motor vehicle administration to find a motor-cycle rider-training course near you.

Practice Operating Your Motorcycle

Given the fact that motorcycles vary in handling and responsive-ness, be sure to take the time to get accustomed to the feel of a new or unfamiliar motorcycle by riding it in a controlled area. Once you feel comfortable with your bike, you can take it into traffic. Make sure you know how to handle your motorcycle in a variety of conditions (e.g., inclement weather or encountering hazards such as slick roads, potholes, and road debris).

Before Every Ride

Check your motorcycle's tire pressure and tread depth, hand and foot brakes, headlights and signal indicators, and fluid levels before you ride. You should also check under the motorcycle for signs of oil or gas leaks. If you are carrying cargo, you should secure and balance the load on the cycle; and adjust the suspension and tire pressure to accommodate the extra weight. If you are carrying a passenger, she or he should mount the motorcycle only after the engine has started; should sit forward as far as possible, directly behind you; and should keep both feet on the foot rests at all times, even when the motorcycle is stopped. Remind your passenger to keep her or his legs and feet away from the muffler. Tell your pas-senger to hold on firmly to your waist, hips, or belt; keep movement to a minimum; and lean at the same time and in the same direction as you do. Do not let your passenger dismount the motorcycle until you say it is safe.

ON THE ROAD
Wear the Proper Protection

If you are ever in a serious motorcycle crash, the best hope you have for protecting your brain is a motorcycle helmet. Always wear a helmet meeting the U.S. Department of Transportation (DOT) Federal Motor Vehicle Safety Standard (FMVSS). Look for the DOT symbol on the outside back of the helmet. Snell and ANSI labels located inside the helmet also show that the helmet meets the standards of those private, nonprofit organizations.

Arms and legs should be completely covered when riding a motorcycle, ideally by wearing leather or heavy denim. In addition to providing protection in a crash, protective gear also helps prevent dehydration. Boots or shoes should be high enough to cover your ankles, while gloves allow for a better grip and help protect your hands in the event of a crash. Wearing brightly colored clothing with reflective material will make you more visible to other vehicle drivers.

Ride Responsibly

Experienced riders know local traffic laws—and they do not take risks. Obey traffic lights, signs, speed limits, and lane markings; ride with the flow of traffic and leave plenty of room between your bike and other vehicles; and always check behind you and the signal before you change lanes. Remember to ride defensively. The majority of multi-vehicle motorcycle crashes generally are caused when other drivers simply do not see the motorcyclist. Proceed cautiously at intersections and yield to pedestrians and other vehicles as appropriate. You can increase your visibility by applying reflective materials to your motorcycle and by keeping your motorcycle's headlights on at all times, even using high beams during the day.

Be Alcohol and Drug Free

Alcohol and drugs, including some prescribed medications, negatively affect your judgment, coordination, balance, throttle control, and ability to shift gears. These substances also impair your alertness and reduce your reaction time. Even when you are fully alert, it is impossible to predict what other vehicles or pedestrians are going to do. Therefore, make sure you are alcohol and drug free when you get on your motorcycle. Otherwise, you will be heading for trouble.

CHOOSE THE RIGHT MOTORCYCLE HELMET

Wearing the right motorcycle helmet can mean the difference between life and death. We know it can also mean the difference between a comfortable and miserable ride. As you search through the many options—online and in stores—we have tips to help you find a safe helmet that fits.

Find Your Fit
SHAPE
Everyone's head is shaped a bit differently, and that's why helmets come in different shape styles—round oval, intermediate oval (the most common), and long oval. While we all generally have between a round and oval shaped head, it is important to determine your actual shape before buying a helmet. Use a mirror, or have a friend look down on your head from the top. Remember to focus on your head shape, not the shape of your face.

SIZE
When measuring your head, use a cloth tape. Start it just above your eyebrows and circle it around the thickest point in the rear of your head. Cross-reference this measurement with a helmet size chart. A helmet that is too loose will move around or will not sit down completely on your head. A correctly sized helmet will be a little tight, providing even pressure around your head without uncomfortable pressure points. It should not move when you shake your head.

STYLE
There are several different categories of helmets, each with different features that correspond to the various types of riding and different types of bikes, as well as various price points and safety features.

Check Safety Ratings
Make sure your helmet has the DOT symbol on the outside back; this means it meets Federal Motor Vehicle Safety Standard (FMVSS) No. 218.

The National Highway Traffic Safety Administration (NHTSA) does not approve helmets, or any other motor vehicle equipment, instead relying on a self-certification process. However, the NHTSA conducts tests on some helmets to make sure they meet standard. While the selection is typically random, they do take into account feedback and complaints from consumers in determining which helmets to test each year. If a helmet does not meet their standard when tested, they can issue a formal recall of the helmet, requiring that it be removed from stores.

Beware of Unsafe Helmets

While all motorcycle helmets sold in the United States are required to meet the federal standard and have the DOT certification label, there are online and brick-and-mortar retailers who sell what are known as "novelty helmets" that do not meet safety standards. There are also fake DOT labels being sold to put on these unsafe helmets.

Novelty helmets are unsafe and will not protect you in the event of a crash. They should not be purchased and should not be worn while operating or riding on a motorcycle. If you are unsure of whether a helmet is unsafe, click below for some tips that can help you identify unsafe helmets.

Section 26.4 | Avoid Impaired Driving

This section contains text excerpted from the following sources: Text beginning with the heading "The Problem" is excerpted from "Impaired Driving: Get the Facts," Centers for Disease Control and Prevention (CDC), March 22, 2019.; Text under the heading "Strategies to Reduce or Prevent Drunk Driving" is excerpted from "What Works: Strategies to Reduce or Prevent Drunk Driving," Centers for Disease Control and Prevention (CDC), March 22, 2016.

THE PROBLEM
How Big Is the Problem?

- In 2016, 10,497 people died in alcohol-impaired driving crashes, accounting for 28 percent of all traffic-related deaths in the United States.
- Of the 1,233 traffic deaths among children 0 to 14 years of age in 2016, 214 (17%) involved an alcohol-impaired driver.

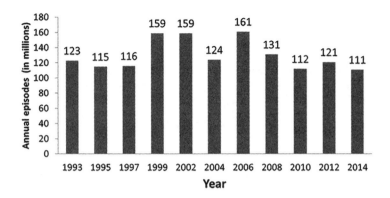

Figure 26.1. Annual Self-Reported Alcohol-Impaired Driving Episodes among U.S. Adults, 1993–2014. *(Source: CDC. Behavioral Risk Factor Surveillance System (BRFSS), 1993–2014.)*

Note: The annual estimated alcohol-impaired driving episodes were calculated using BRFSS respondents' answers to this question: "During the past 30 days, how many times have you driven when you have had perhaps too much to drink?" Annual estimates per respondent were calculated by multiplying the reported episodes during the preceding 30 days by 12. These numbers were summed to obtain the annual national estimates (see www.cdc.gov/mmwr/preview/mmwrhtml/mm6430a2.htm).

- In 2016, more than 1 million drivers were arrested for driving under the influence of alcohol or narcotics. That is one percent of the 111 million self-reported episodes of alcohol-impaired driving among U.S. adults each year.
- Drugs other than alcohol (legal and illegal) are involved in about 16 percent of motor vehicle crashes.
- Marijuana use is increasing and 13 percent of nighttime, weekend drivers have marijuana in their system.
- Marijuana users are about 25 percent more likely to be involved in a crash than drivers with no evidence of marijuana use, however other factors—such as age and gender—may account for the increased crash risk among marijuana users.

RISK FACTORS
Who Is Most at Risk?

Young people:

- At all levels of blood alcohol concentration (BAC), the risk of being involved in a crash is greater for young people than for older people.
- Among drivers with BAC levels of 0.08 percent or higher involved in fatal crashes in 2016, nearly three in 10 were between 25 and 34 years of age (27%). The next two largest groups were ages 21 to 24 (26%) and 35 to 44 years of age (22%).

Motorcyclists:

- Among motorcyclists killed in fatal crashes in 2016, 25 percent had BACs of 0.08 percent or greater.
- Motorcyclists 35 to 39 years of age have the highest percentage of deaths with BACs of 0.08 percent or greater (38% in 2016).

Drivers with prior driving while impaired (driving while intoxicated (DWI) convictions:

- Drivers with a BAC of 0.08 percent or higher involved in fatal crashes were 4.5 times more likely to have a prior conviction for DWI than were drivers with no alcohol in their system. (9% and 2%, respectively).

BLOOD ALCOHOL CONCENTRATION EFFECTS
What Are the Effects of Blood Alcohol Concentration?

Information in this table shows the blood alcohol concentration (BAC) level at which the effect usually is first observed.

PREVENTION
How Can Deaths and Injuries from Impaired Driving Be Prevented?

Effective measures include:

- Actively enforcing existing 0.08 percent BAC laws, minimum legal drinking age laws, and zero tolerance

Table 26.1. Blood Alcohol Concentration and Its Effects

Blood Alcohol Concentration (BAC)*	Typical Effects	Predictable Effects on Driving
0.02 percent About 2 alcoholic drinks**	• Some loss of judgment • Relaxation • Slight body warmth • Altered mood	• Decline in visual functions (rapid tracking of a moving target) • Decline in ability to perform two tasks at the same time (divided attention)
0.05 percent About 3 alcoholic drinks**	• Exaggerated behavior • May have loss of small-muscle control (e.g., focusing your eyes) • Impaired judgment • Usually good feeling • Lowered alertness • Release of inhibition	• Reduced coordination • Reduced ability to track moving objects • Difficulty steering • Reduced response to emergency driving situations
0.08 percent About 4 alcoholic drinks**	• Muscle coordination becomes poor (e.g., balance, speech, vision, reaction time, and hearing) • Harder to detect danger • Judgment, self-control, reasoning, and memory are impaired	• Concentration • Short-term memory loss • Speed control • Reduced information processing capability (e.g., signal detection, visual search) • Impaired perception
0.10 percent About 5 alcoholic drinks**	• Clear deterioration of reaction time and control • Slurred speech, poor coordination, and slowed thinking	• Reduced ability to maintain lane position and brake appropriately
0.15 percent About 7 alcoholic drinks**	• Far less muscle control than normal • Vomiting may occur (unless this level is reached slowly or a person has developed a tolerance for alcohol) • Major loss of balance	• Substantial impairment in vehicle control, attention to driving task, and in necessary visual and auditory information processing

*Blood Alcohol Concentration Measurement
The number of drinks listed represents the approximate amount of alcohol that a 160-pound man would need to drink in one hour to reach the listed BAC in each category.
**A Standard Drink Size in the United States
A standard drink is equal to 14.0 grams (0.6 ounces) of pure alcohol. Generally, this amount of pure alcohol is found in:
• 12-ounces of beer (5% alcohol content)
• 8-ounces of malt liquor (7% alcohol content)
• 5-ounces of wine (12% alcohol content)
• 1.5-ounces or a "shot" of 80-proof (40% alcohol content) distilled spirits or liquor (e.g., gin, rum, vodka, whiskey)

laws for drivers younger than 21 years of age in all states
- Requiring ignition interlocks for all offenders, including first-time offenders
- Using sobriety checkpoints
- Putting health promotion efforts into practice that influence economic, organizational, policy, and school/community action
- Using community-based approaches to alcohol control and DWI prevention
- Requiring mandatory substance abuse assessment and treatment, if needed, for DWI offenders
- Raising the unit price of alcohol by increasing taxes

What Safety Steps Can Individuals Take?

Whenever your social plans involve alcohol and/or drugs, make plans so that you do not have to drive while impaired. For example:
- Before drinking, designate a nondrinking driver when with a group.
- Do not let your friends drive impaired.
- If you have been drinking or using drugs, get a ride home, use a rideshare service or call a taxi.
- If you are hosting a party where alcohol will be served, remind your guests to plan ahead and designate their sober driver; offer alcohol-free beverages, and make sure all guests leave with a sober driver.

STRATEGIES TO REDUCE OR PREVENT DRUNK DRIVING

The strategies in this section are effective for reducing or preventing drunk driving. They are recommended by The Guide to Community Preventive Services and/or have been demonstrated to be effective in reviews by the National Highway Traffic Safety Administration. Different strategies may require different resources for implementation or have different levels of impact. Find strategies that are right for your state.

Drunk Driving Laws

Drunk driving laws make it illegal nationwide to drive with a BAC at or above 0.08 percent. For people under 21, "zero tolerance" laws make it illegal to drive with any measurable amount of alcohol in their system. These laws, along with laws that maintain the minimum legal drinking age at 21, are in place in all 50 states and the District of Columbia, and have had a clear effect on highway safety, saving tens of thousands of lives since their implementation.

Sobriety Checkpoints

Sobriety checkpoints allow police to briefly stop vehicles at specific, highly visible locations to see if the driver is impaired. Police may stop all or a certain portion of drivers. Breath tests may be given if police have a reason to suspect the driver is intoxicated.

Ignition Interlocks

Ignition interlocks installed in cars measure alcohol on the driver's breath. Interlocks keep the car from starting if the driver has a BAC above a certain level, usually 0.02 percent. They're used for people convicted of drunk driving and are highly effective at preventing repeat offenses while installed. Mandating interlocks for all offenders, including first-time offenders, will have the greatest impact.

Multi-Component Interventions

Multi-component interventions combine several programs or policies to prevent drunk driving. The key to these comprehensive efforts is community mobilization by involving coalitions or task forces in design and implementation.

Mass Media Campaigns

Mass media campaigns spread messages about the physical dangers and legal consequences of drunk driving. They persuade people not to drink and drive and encourage them to keep other drivers from doing so. Campaigns are most effective when supporting other impaired driving prevention strategies.

Administrative License Revocation or Suspension Laws

Administrative license revocation or suspension laws allow police to take away the license of a driver who tests at or above the legal BAC limit or who refuses testing. States decide how long to suspend the license; a minimum of 90 days is effective.

Alcohol Screening and Brief Interventions

Alcohol screening and brief interventions take advantage of "teachable moments" to identify people at risk for alcohol problems and get them treatment as needed. This combined strategy, which can be delivered in healthcare, university, and other settings, helps change behavior and reduces alcohol-impaired crashes and injuries.

School-Based Instructional Programs

School-based instructional programs are effective at teaching teens not to ride with drunk drivers. More evidence is needed to see if these programs can also reduce drunk driving and related crashes.

Section 26.5 | Refrain from Distracted Driving

This section includes text excerpted from "Distracted Driving," National Highway Traffic Safety Administration (NHTSA), April 1, 2020.

Distracted driving is dangerous, claiming 2,841 lives in 2018 alone. Among those killed: 1,730 drivers, 605 passengers, 400 pedestrians, and 77 bicyclists. The National Highway Traffic Safety Administration (NHTSA) leads the national effort to save lives by preventing this dangerous behavior. Get the facts, get involved, and help the National Highway Traffic Safety Administration (NHTSA) to keep America's roads safe.

WHAT IS DISTRACTED DRIVING?

Distracted driving is any activity that diverts attention from driving, including talking or texting on your phone, eating and drinking, talking to people in your vehicle, fiddling with the stereo, entertainment, or navigation system—anything that takes your attention away from the task of safe driving. Texting is the most alarming distraction. Sending or reading a text takes your eyes off the road for 5 seconds. At 55 mph, that is like driving the length of an entire football field with your eyes closed. You cannot drive safely unless the task of driving has your full attention. Any nondriving activity you engage in is a potential distraction and increases your risk of crashing.

CONSEQUENCES

Using a cell phone while driving creates enormous potential for deaths and injuries on U.S. roads. In 2018 alone, 2,841 people were killed in motor vehicle crashes involving distracted drivers.

GET INVOLVED

Everyone can all play a part in the fight to save lives by ending distracted driving.

Teens

Teens can be the best messengers with their peers, so the NHTSA encourages them to speak up when they see a friend driving while distracted, to have their friends sign a pledge to never drive distracted, to become involved in their local Students Against Destructive Decisions (SADD) chapter, and to share messages on social media that remind their friends, family, and neighbors not to make the deadly choice of distracted driving.

Parents

Parents first have to lead by example—by never driving distracted—as well as have a talk with their young driver about distraction and all of the responsibilities that come with driving. Have everyone in the family sign the pledge to commit to distraction-free driving. Remind your teen driver that in states with graduated driver licensing (GDL), a violation of distracted-driving laws could mean a delayed or suspended license.

Educators and Employers

Educators and employers can play a part, too. Spread the word at your school or workplace about the dangers of distracted driving. Ask your students to commit to distraction-free driving or set a company policy on distracted driving.

Make Your Voice Heard

If you feel strongly about distracted driving, be a voice in your community by supporting local laws, speaking out at community meetings, and highlighting the dangers of distracted driving on social media and in your local op-ed pages.

Section 26.6 | Pedestrian Safety

This section includes text excerpted from "Pedestrian Safety," National Highway Traffic Safety Administration (NHTSA), November 5, 2018.

WALKING SAFETY TIPS

- Be predictable. Follow the rules of the road and obey signs and signals.
- Walk on sidewalks whenever they are available.
- If there is no sidewalk, walk facing traffic and as far from traffic as possible.
- Keep alert at all times; do not be distracted by electronic devices that take your eyes (and ears) off the road.
- Whenever possible, cross streets at crosswalks or intersections, where drivers expect pedestrians. Look for cars in all directions, including those turning left or right.
- If a crosswalk or intersection is not available, locate a well-lit area where you have the best view of traffic. Wait for a gap in traffic that allows enough time to cross safely; continue watching for traffic as you cross.
- Never assume a driver sees you. Make eye contact with drivers as they approach to make sure you are seen.

- Be visible at all times. Wear bright clothing during the day, and wear reflective materials or use a flashlight at night.
- Watch for cars entering or exiting driveways, or backing up in parking lots.
- Avoid alcohol and drugs when walking; they impair your abilities and your judgment.

DRIVING SAFETY TIPS

- Look out for pedestrians everywhere, at all times. Safety is a shared responsibility.
- Use extra caution when driving in hard-to-see conditions, such as nighttime or bad weather.
- Slow down and be prepared to stop when turning or otherwise entering a crosswalk.
- Yield to pedestrians in crosswalks and stop well back from the crosswalk to give other vehicles an opportunity to see the crossing pedestrians so they can stop too.
- Never pass vehicles stopped at a crosswalk. There may be people crossing whom you cannot see.
- Never drive under the influence of alcohol and/or drugs.
- Follow the speed limit, especially around people on the street.
- Follow slower speed limits in school zones and in neighborhoods where children are present.
- Be extra cautious when backing up—pedestrians can move into your path.

Section 26.7 | **School Bus Safety**

This section includes text excerpted from "School Bus Safety," National Highway Traffic Safety Administration (NHTSA), October 16, 2014. Reviewed May 2020.

BUS SAFETY

Students are about 70 times more likely to get to school safely when taking a bus instead of traveling by car. That is because school buses are the most regulated vehicles on the road; they are designed to be safer than passenger vehicles in preventing crashes and injuries; and in every state, stop-arm laws protect children from other motorists.

- **Different by Design.** School buses are designed so that they are highly visible and include safety features such as flashing red lights, cross-view mirrors, and stop-sign arms. They also include protective seating, high crush standards, and rollover protection features.
- **Protected by the Law.** Laws protect students who are getting off and on a school bus by making it illegal for drivers to pass a school bus while dropping off or picking up passengers, regardless of the direction of approach.

Seat Belts on School Buses

Seat belts have been required on passenger cars since 1968, and 49 states and the District of Columbia have enacted laws requiring the use of seat belts in passenger cars and light trucks. There is no question that seat belts play an important role in keeping passengers safe in these vehicles. But, school buses are different by design, including a different kind of safety restraint system that works extremely well.

Large school buses are heavier and distribute crash forces differently than passenger cars and light trucks do. Because of these differences, bus passengers experience much less crash force than those in passenger cars, light trucks, and vans.

The National Highway Traffic Safety Administration (NHTSA) decided that the best way to provide crash protection to passengers of large school buses is through a concept called "compartmentalization." This requires that the interior of large buses protect children without them needing to buckle up. Through compartmentalization, children are protected from crashes by strong, closely-spaced seats that have energy-absorbing seat backs.

Small school buses (with a gross vehicle weight rating of 10,000 pounds or less) must be equipped with lap and/or lap/shoulder belts at all designated seating positions. Since the sizes and weights of small school buses are closer to those of passenger cars and trucks, seat belts in those vehicles are necessary to provide occupant protection.

BUS STOP SAFETY

The greatest risk to your child is not riding a bus, but approaching or leaving one. Before your child goes back to school or starts school for the first time, it is important for you and your child to know traffic safety rules. Teach your child to follow these practices to make school bus transportation safer.

For Parents
SAFETY STARTS AT THE BUS STOP

Your child should arrive at the bus stop at least five minutes before the bus is scheduled to arrive. Visit the bus stop and show your child where to wait for the bus: at least three giant steps (six feet) away from the curb. Remind your child that the bus stop is not a place to run or play.

GET ON AND OFF SAFELY

When the school bus arrives, your child should wait until the bus comes to a complete stop, the door opens, and the driver says it is okay before approaching the bus door. Your child should use the handrails to avoid falling.

USE CAUTION AROUND THE BUS

Your child should never walk behind a school bus. If your child must cross the street in front of the bus, tell her or him to walk on a sidewalk or along the side of the street to a place at least five giant steps (10 feet) in front of the bus before crossing. Your child should also make eye contact with the bus driver before crossing to make sure the driver can see her or him. If your child drops something near the school bus, like a ball or book, the safest thing is for your child to tell the bus driver right away. Your child should not try to pick up the item, because the driver might not be able to see her or him.

For Drivers

Make school bus transportation safer for everyone by following these practices:

- When backing out of a driveway or leaving a garage, watch out for children walking or bicycling to school.
- When driving in neighborhoods with school zones, watch out for young people who may be thinking about getting to school, but may not be thinking of getting there safely.
- Slow down. Watch for children walking in the street, especially if there are no sidewalks in neighborhood.
- Watch for children playing and congregating near bus stops.
- Be alert. Children arriving late for the bus may dart into the street without looking for traffic.
- Learn and obey the school bus laws in your state, as well as the "flashing signal light system" that school bus drivers use to alert motorists of pending actions:
  - **Yellow flashing lights** indicate the bus is preparing to stop to load or unload children. Motorists should slow down and prepare to stop their vehicles.
  - **Red flashing lightsand extended stop arms** indicate the bus has stopped and children are getting on or off. Motorists must stop their cars and wait until the red lights stop flashing, the extended stop-arm is withdrawn, and the bus begins moving before they can start driving again.
- School Bus Driver In-Service Safety Series. This refresher training provides nine-lesson modules on

driving a school bus, which is frequently requested by
school bus drivers and pupil transportation supervisors.

Section 26.8 | Teen Driving Safety

This section contains text excerpted from the following sources: Text in this section begins with excerpts
from "Teen Drivers: Get the Facts," Centers for Disease Control and Prevention (CDC), October 30, 2019;
Text under the heading "Eight Danger Zones: Prevention" is excerpted from "Eight Danger Zones," Centers
for Disease Control and Prevention (CDC), October 4, 2019; Text under the heading "Graduated Driver
Licensing" is excerpted from "Eight Danger Zones," Centers for Disease Control and Prevention (CDC),
December 20, 2016. Reviewed May 2020; Text under the heading "Parent-Teen Driving Agreement" is
excerpted from "Parent-Teen Driving Agreement," Centers for Disease Control and Prevention (CDC),
October 14, 2016. Reviewed May 2020;

Motor vehicle crashes are the leading cause of death for U.S. teens.
Teen motor vehicle crashes are preventable, and proven strategies
can improve the safety of young drivers on the road.

THE PROBLEM
How Big Is the Problem?

In 2017, 2,364 teens in the United States 16 to 19 years of age were
killed, and about 300,000 were treated in emergency departments
(ED) for injuries suffered in motor vehicle crashes. That means
six teens 16 to 19 years of age died every day due to motor vehicle
crashes, and hundreds more were injured.

In 2017, young people 15 to 19 years of age represented 6.5
percent of the U.S. population. However, motor vehicle injuries,
both fatal and nonfatal, among young people in this age group
represented about $13.1 billion, or almost 8 percent, of the total
costs of motor vehicle injuries.

RISK GROUPS
Who Is Most at Risk?

The risk of motor vehicle crashes is higher among teens 16 to 19
years of age than among any other age group. In fact, per mile

driven, teen drivers in this age group are nearly three times more likely than drivers 20 years of age and older to be in a fatal crash.

Teens who are at especially high risk for motor vehicle crashes are:

- Male
  - In 2017, the motor vehicle death rate for male drivers 16 to 19 years of age was over two times higher than the death rate for female drivers of the same age.
- Teens driving with teen passengers
  - The presence of teen passengers increases the crash risk of unsupervised teen drivers. This risk increases with increased numbers of teen passengers.
- Newly licensed teens
  - Crash risk is particularly high during the first months of licensure. Data from the 2017 National Household Travel Survey (NHTS) indicate that the crash rate per mile driven is 1.5 times higher for 16-year-olds than it is for 18 to 19 year-olds.

RISK FACTORS
What Factors Put Teen Drivers at Risk?

- Inexperience
  - Teens are more likely than older drivers to underestimate or not be able to recognize dangerous situations. Teens are also more likely than adults to make critical decision errors that lead to serious crashes.
- Speeding
  - Teens are more likely than older drivers to speed and allow shorter headways (the distance from the front of one vehicle to the front of the next).
- Seat belt use
  - Compared with other age groups, teens and young adults often have the lowest seat belt use rates. In 2017, only 58.8 percent of high school students always wore seat belts when riding as passengers.

- Among young drivers 15 to 20 years of age who died in car crashes in 2017, almost half were unrestrained at the time of the crash (when restraint use was known).
- Alcohol use
  - Any amount of alcohol increases the risk of crashes among teens as compared with older drivers.
  - In the 2017 national Youth Risk Behavior Survey (YRBS), 16.5 percent of high school students had ridden with a driver who had been drinking alcohol within the previous month. Among students who drove, 5.5 percent drove when they had been drinking alcohol during the 30 days before the survey.
  - Drinking alcohol is illegal under 21 years of age; therefore, so is drinking and driving. Despite this, in 2017, 15 percent of drivers 16 to 20 years of age involved in fatal motor vehicle crashes had a blood alcohol concentration (BAC) of .08 percent or higher (a level that is illegal for adults 21 years of age and older in all states, except Utah, which has a BAC limit of .05).
  - In 2017, 58 percent of drivers 15 to 20 years of age who were killed in motor vehicle crashes after drinking and driving were not wearing a seat belt (based on known restraint use).
  - Among male drivers 15 to 20 years of age who were involved in fatal crashes in 2017, 31 percent were speeding at the time of the crash 17 and 20 percent had been drinking.
- Nighttime and weekend driving
  - In 2017, 40 percent of motor vehicle crash deaths among teen drivers and passengers 13- to 19 occurred between 9 p.m. and 6 a.m., and 51 percent occurred on Friday, Saturday, or Sunday.

EIGHT DANGER ZONES: PREVENTION

Six teens a day are killed in car crashes. But, injuries and deaths are preventable. Make sure your young driver is aware of the leading causes of teen crashes. Then use a parent-teen driving agreement to put rules in place that will help your teen stay safe.

Danger Zone #1: Driver Inexperience
Crash risk is highest in the first year a teen has their license.

WHAT PARENTS CAN DO
- Provide at least 30 to 50 hours of supervised driving practice over at least six months.
- Practice on a variety of roads, at different times of day, and in varied weather and traffic conditions.
- Stress the importance of continually scanning for potential hazards including other vehicles, bicyclists, and pedestrians.

Danger Zone #2: Driving with Teen Passengers
Crash risk goes up when teens drive with other teens in the car.

WHAT PARENTS CAN DO
- Follow your state's Graduated Driver Licensing (GDL) system for passenger restrictions. If your state does not have such a rule, limit the number of teen passengers your teen can have to zero or one.
- Keep this rule for at least the first six months that your teen is driving.

Danger Zone #3: Nighttime Driving
For all ages, fatal crashes are more likely to occur at night; but the risk is higher for teens.

WHAT PARENTS CAN DO
- Make sure your teen is off the road by 9 or 10 p.m. for at least the first six months of licensed driving.
- Practice nighttime driving with your teen when you think they are ready.

Danger Zone #4: Not Using Seat Belts

The simplest way to prevent car crash deaths is to buckle up.

WHAT PARENTS CAN DO

- Require your teen to wear a seat belt on every trip. This simple step can reduce your teen's risk of dying or being badly injured in a crash by about half.

Danger Zone #5: Distracted Driving

Distractions increase your teen's risk of being in a crash.

WHAT PARENTS CAN DO

- Do not allow activities that may take your teen's attention away from driving such as talking on a cell phone, texting, eating, or playing with the radio.
- Learn more about distracted driving.

Danger Zone #6: Drowsy Driving

Young drivers are at high risk for drowsy driving, which causes thousands of crashes every year. Teens are most tired and at risk when driving in the early morning or late at night.

WHAT PARENTS CAN DO

- Know your teen's schedule so you can be sure she or he is well-rested before getting behind the wheel.

Danger Zone #7: Reckless Driving

Research shows that teens lack the experience, judgment, and maturity to assess risky situations.

WHAT PARENTS CAN DO

- Make sure your teen knows to follow the speed limit and adjust their speed to match road conditions.

- Remind your teen to maintain enough space behind the vehicle ahead to avoid a crash in case of a sudden stop.

Danger Zone #8: Impaired Driving

Even one drink will impair your teen's driving ability and increase their risk of a crash.

WHAT PARENTS CAN DO

- Be a good role model: never drink and drive.
- Reinforce this message with a Parent-Teen Driving Agreement.

GRADUATED DRIVER LICENSING

Graduated Driver Licensing (GDL) systems help new drivers gain skills under lower-risk conditions. As drivers move through the three stages of GDL, they are given more driving privileges. These privileges may include driving at night or with passengers. GDL systems are proven to reduce teen crashes and deaths.

All states have three-stage GDL systems, though laws vary.

- Stage 1: Learner's permit
- Stage 2: Intermediate license (sometimes called a "provisional license")
- Stage 3: Unrestricted license

PARENT-TEEN DRIVING AGREEMENT

Having regular conversations about safety, practicing driving together, and leading by example go a long way in ensuring your teen makes smart decisions when they get behind the wheel.

But, there is another simple step you can take to get on the same page about your family's rules of the road. Create a Parent-Teen Driving Agreement that puts your rules in writing to clearly set expectations and limits. Work with your teen to outline hazards to avoid and consequences for breaking rules. Keep it on the fridge and update it as your teen gains experience and more driving privileges.

Section 26.9 | **Aging and Driving**

This section includes text excerpted from "Older Drivers," National Institute on Aging (NIA), National Institutes of Health (NIH), December 12, 2018.

STIFF JOINTS AND MUSCLES

As you age, your joints may get stiff, and your muscles may weaken. Arthritis, which is common among older adults, might affect your ability to drive. These changes can make it harder to turn your head to look back, turn the steering wheel quickly, or brake safely.

Safe driving tips:

- See your doctor if pain, stiffness, or arthritis seem to get in the way of your driving.
- If possible, drive a car with automatic transmission, power steering, power brakes, and large mirrors.
- Be physically active or exercise to improve your strength and flexibility.
- Think about getting hand controls for both the gas and brake pedals if you have leg problems.

TROUBLE SEEING

Your eyesight can change as you get older. It might be harder to see people, things, and movement outside your direct line of sight. It may take longer to read street or traffic signs or even recognize familiar places. At night, you may have trouble seeing things clearly. Glare from oncoming headlights or street lights can be a problem. Depending on the time of the day, the sun might be blinding.

Eye diseases such as glaucoma, cataracts, and macular degeneration, as well as some medicines, can also cause vision problems.

Safe driving tips:

- If you are 65 years of age or older, see your eye doctor every year. Ask if there are ways to improve your eyesight.
- If you need glasses or contact lenses to see far away while driving, make sure your prescription is up-to-date and correct. Always wear them when you are driving.

- Cut back on or stop driving at night if you have trouble seeing in the dark. Try to avoid driving during sunrise and sunset, when the sun can be directly in your line of vision.

TROUBLE HEARING

As you get older, your hearing can change, making it harder to notice horns, sirens, or even noises coming from your own car. Hearing loss can be a problem because these sounds warn you when you may need to pull over or get out of the way.

Safe driving tips:

- Have your hearing checked at least every 3 years after 50 years of age.
- Discuss concerns you have about hearing with your doctor. There may be things that can help.
- Try to keep the inside of the car as quiet as possible while driving.

Dementia and Driving

In the very early stages of Alzheimer disease (AD) or other types of dementia, some people are able to keep driving. But, as memory and decision-making skills get worse, they need to stop.

People with dementia often do not know they are having driving problems. Family and friends need to monitor the person's driving ability and take action as soon as they observe a potential problem, such as forgetting how to find familiar places like the grocery store or even their home. Work with the doctor to let the person know it is no longer safe to keep driving.

SLOWER REACTION TIME AND REFLEXES

As you get older, your reflexes might get slower, and you might not react as quickly as you could in the past. You might find that you have a shorter attention span, making it harder to do two things at once. Stiff joints or weak muscles also can make it harder to move quickly. Loss of feeling or tingling in your fingers and feet can make it difficult to steer or use the foot pedals. Parkinson disease

(PD) or limitations following a stroke can make it no longer safe to drive.

Safe driving tips:

- Leave more space between you and the car in front of you.
- Start braking early when you need to stop.
- Avoid heavy traffic areas or rush-hour driving when you can.
- If you must drive on a fast-moving highway, drive in the right-hand lane. Traffic moves more slowly there, giving you more time to make safe driving decisions.

MEDICATIONS CAN AFFECT DRIVING

Do you take any medicines that make you feel drowsy, lightheaded, or less alert than usual? Do medicines you take have a warning about driving? Many medications have side effects that can make driving unsafe. Pay attention to how these drugs may affect your driving.

Safe driving tips:

- Read medicine labels carefully. Look for any warnings.
- Make a list of all of your medicines, and talk with your doctor or pharmacist about how they can affect your driving.
- Do not drive if you feel lightheaded or drowsy.

BE A SAFE DRIVER

Maybe you already know that driving at night, on the highway, or in bad weather is a problem for you. Some older drivers also have problems when yielding the right of way, turning (especially making left turns), changing lanes, passing, and using expressway ramps.

Safe driving tips:

- Have your driving skills checked by a driving rehabilitation specialist, occupational therapist, or other trained professional.
- Take a defensive driving course. Some car insurance companies may lower your bill when you pass this type

of class. Organizations such as American Association of Retired Persons (AARP), American Automobile Association (AAA), or your car insurance company can help you find a class near you.

- When in doubt, do not go out. Bad weather such as rain, ice, or snow can make it hard for anyone to drive. Try to wait until the weather is better, or use buses, taxis, or other transportation services.
- Avoid areas where driving can be a problem. For example, choose a route that avoids highways or other high-speed roadways. Or, find a way to go that requires few or no left turns.
- Ask your doctor if any of your health problems or medications might make it unsafe for you to drive. Together, you can make a plan to help you keep driving and decide when it is no longer safe to drive.

DO YOU HAVE CONCERNS ABOUT AN OLDER DRIVER?

Are you worried about an older family member or friend driving? Sometimes, it can be hard for an older person to realize that she or he is no longer a safe driver. You might want to observe the person's driving skills.

If it is not possible to observe the older person driving, look out for these signs:

- Multiple vehicle crashes, "near misses," and/or new dents in the car
- Two or more traffic tickets or warnings within the last two years; increases in car insurance premiums because of driving issues
- Comments from neighbors or friends about driving
- Anxiety about driving at night
- Health issues that might affect driving ability, including problems with vision, hearing, and/or movement
- Complaints about the speed, sudden lane changes, or actions of other drivers
- Recommendations from a doctor to modify driving habits or quit driving entirely

Having "The Talk" about Driving

Talking with an older person about her or his driving is often difficult. Here are some things that might help when having the talk.

- **Be prepared.** Learn about local services to help someone who can no longer drive. Identify the person's transportation needs.
- **Avoid confrontation.** Use "I" messages rather than "You" messages. For example, say, "I am concerned about your safety when you are driving," rather than, "You're no longer a safe driver."
- **Stick to the issue**. Discuss the driver's skills, not her or his age.
- **Focus on safety and maintaining independence.** Be clear that the goal is for the older driver to continue the activities she or he currently enjoys while staying safe. Offer to help the person stay independent. For example, you might say, "I'll help you figure out how to get where you want to go if driving isn't possible."
- **Be positive and supportive.** Recognize the importance of a driver's license to the older person. Understand that she or he may become defensive, angry, hurt, or withdrawn. You might say, "I understand that this may be upsetting" or "We'll work together to find a solution."

IS IT TIME TO GIVE UP DRIVING?

We all age differently. For this reason, there is no way to set one age when everyone should stop driving. So, how do you know if you should stop? To help decide, ask yourself:

- Do other drivers often honk at me?
- Have I had some accidents, even if they were only "fender benders"?
- Do I get lost, even on roads I know?
- Do cars or people walking seem to appear out of nowhere?
- Do I get distracted while driving?
- Have family, friends, or my doctor said they are worried about my driving?

- Am I driving less these days because I'm not as sure about my driving as I used to be?
- Do I have trouble staying in my lane?
- Do I have trouble moving my foot between the gas and the brake pedals, or do I sometimes confuse the two?
- Have I been pulled over by a police officer about my driving?

If you answered "yes" to any of these questions, it may be time to talk with your doctor about driving or have a driving assessment.

HOW WILL YOU GET AROUND?

Are you worried you will not be able to do the things you want and need to do if you stop driving? Many people have this concern, but there may be more ways to get around than you think. For example, some areas provide free or low-cost bus or taxi services for older people. Some communities offer a carpool service or scheduled trips to the grocery store, mall, or doctor's office. Religious and civic groups sometimes have volunteers who will drive you where you want to go.

Your local Area Agency on Aging (AAA) can help you find services in your area. Call 800-677-1116, or go to eldercare.acl.gov to find your nearest AAA.

You can also think about using a car or ride-sharing service. Sound pricey? Do not forget—it costs a lot to own a car. If you do not have to make car payments or pay for insurance, maintenance, gas, oil, or other car expenses, then you may be able to afford to take taxis or other transportation. You can also buy gas for friends or family members who give you rides.

More Safe Driving Tips

Before you leave home:
- Plan to drive on streets you know
- Only drive to places that are easy to get to and close to home
- Avoid risky spots like ramps and left turns

Stay Safe on Roads

- Add extra time for travel if you must drive when conditions are poor
- Limit how much you drive at night
- Do not drive when you are stressed or tired

While you are driving:
- Always wear your seat belt and make sure your passengers wear their seat belts, too
- Wear your glasses and/or hearing aid, if you use them
- Stay off your cell phone
- Avoid distractions such as eating, listening to the radio, or chatting
- Use your window defrosters to keep both the front and back windows clear

Chapter 27 | **Workplace Safety**

Falls are a hazard found in many work settings. A fall can occur during walking or climbing a ladder to change a light fixture, or as a result of a complex series of events affecting an ironworker 80 feet above the ground.

JOB HAZARDS
Circumstances associated with fall incidents in the work environment frequently involve:
- Slippery, cluttered, or unstable walking/working surfaces
- Unprotected edges
- Floor holes and wall openings
- Unsafely positioned ladders
- Misused fall protection

HOW BIG OF AN ISSUE ARE FALLS IN THE WORKPLACE?
Based on 2014 published data from the Bureau of Labor Statistics (BLS), 261,930 private industry and state and local government workers missed one or more days of work due to injuries from falls on the same level or to lower levels, and 798 workers died from such falls.

This chapter contains text excerpted from the following sources: Text in this chapter begins with excerpts from "Falls in the Workplace," Centers for Disease Control and Prevention (CDC), October 2, 2019; Text under the heading "What Can Be Done to Reduce Falls?" is excerpted from "Fall Protection—Safety and Health Topics," Occupational Safety and Health Administration (OSHA), April 3, 2012. Reviewed May 2020; Text under the heading "OSHA's Fall Prevention Campaign" is excerpted from "Welcome to OSHA's Fall Prevention Campaign," National Institutes of Allergy and Infectious Diseases (NIAID), September 16, 2013. Reviewed May 2020.

The construction industry experienced the highest frequency of fall-related deaths, while the highest counts of nonfatal fall injuries continue to be associated with the health services and the wholesale and retail industries. Particularly at risk of fall injuries are those working in:

- Healthcare support
- Building cleaning and maintenance
- Transportation and material moving
- Construction and extraction occupations

Fall injuries create a considerable financial burden: workers' compensation and medical costs associated with occupational fall incidents have been estimated at $70 billion annually in the United States. Many other countries face similar challenges in the workplace. In fact, the international public-health community has a strong interest in developing strategies to reduce the toll of fall injuries.

WHAT CAN BE DONE TO REDUCE FALLS?

Employers must set up the workplace to prevent employees from falling off of overhead platforms, elevated work stations, or holes in the floor and walls. The Occupational Safety and Health Administration (OSHA) requires that fall protection be provided at elevations of four feet in general industry workplaces, five feet in shipyards, six feet in the construction industry, and eight feet in longshoring operations. In addition, OSHA requires that fall protection be provided when working over dangerous equipment and machinery, regardless of the fall distance.

To prevent employees from being injured from falls, employers must:

- Guard every floor hole (using a railing and toe-board or a floor hole cover) into which a worker can accidentally walk.
- Provide a guard rail and toe-board around every elevated open sided platform, floor, or runway.
- Regardless of height, if a worker can fall into or onto dangerous machines or equipment (such as a vat of acid or a conveyor belt) employers must provide

guardrails and toe-boards to prevent workers from falling and getting injured.
- Other means of fall protection that may be required on certain jobs include safety harness and line, safety nets, stair railings, and handrails.

OSHA requires employers to:
- Provide working conditions that are free of known dangers.
- Keep floors in work areas in a clean and, as far as possible, a dry condition.
- Select and provide required personal protective equipment at no cost to workers.
- Train workers about job hazards in a language that they can understand.

OSHA'S FALL PREVENTION CAMPAIGN

Since 2012, OSHA has partnered with the National Institute for Occupational Safety and Health and National Occupational Research Agenda (NORA)-Construction Sector on the Fall Prevention Campaign to raise awareness among workers and employers about common fall hazards in construction, and how falls from ladders, scaffolds, and roofs can be prevented.

Plan Ahead to Get the Job Done Safely

When working from heights, employers must plan projects to ensure that the job is done safely. Begin by deciding how the job will be done, what tasks will be involved, and what safety equipment may be needed to complete each task.

When estimating the cost of a job, employers should include safety equipment and plan to have all the necessary equipment and tools available at the construction site. For example, in a roofing job, think about all of the different fall hazards, such as holes or skylights and leading edges, then plan and select fall protection suitable to that work, such as personal fall arrest systems (PFAS).

Provide the Right Equipment

Workers who are six feet or more above lower levels are at risk for serious injury or death if they should fall. To protect these workers, employers must provide fall protection and the right equipment for the job, including the right kinds of ladders, scaffolds, and safety gear.

Use the right ladder or scaffold to get the job done safely. For roof work, if workers use PFAS, provide a harness for each worker who needs to tie off to the anchor. Make sure the PFAS fits, and regularly inspect it for safe use.

Train Everyone to Use the Equipment Safely

Every worker should be trained on proper setup and safe use of equipment they use on the job. Employers must train workers in recognizing hazards on the job.

Chapter 28 | **Playground Safety**

Each year in the United States, emergency departments (EDs) treat more than 200,000 children ages 14 and younger for playground-related injuries. More than 20,000 of these children are treated for a traumatic brain injury (TBI), including concussion. Overall, more research is needed to better understand what specific activities are putting kids at risk of injury and what changes in playground equipment and surfaces might help prevent injuries.

OCCURRENCE AND CONSEQUENCES OF PLAYGROUND-RELATED INJURIES
All Emergency Department-Treated, Playground-Related Injuries
- About 56 percent of playground-related injuries that are treated in EDs are fractures and contusions/abrasions.
- About 75 percent of injuries related to playground equipment occur on public playgrounds. Most occur at a place of recreation or school.

Playground-Related Traumatic Brain Injury
- The overall rate of ED visits for playground-related TBI has significantly increased in recent years (2005–2013).

This chapter contains text excerpted from the following sources: Text in this chapter begins with excerpts from "Playground Safety," Centers for Disease Control and Prevention (CDC), February 6, 2019; Text under the heading "Public Playground Safety Checklist" is excerpted from "Public Playground Safety Checklist," U.S. Consumer Product Safety Commission (CPSC), February 1, 2001. Reviewed May 2020.

- About two-thirds of playground-related TBIs occurred at school and places or recreation or sports and often involved monkey bars, climbing equipment, or swings.
- Most ED visits for playground-related TBIs occur during weekdays, Monday through Friday.
- Playground-related TBI ED visits occurred frequently during the months of April, May, and September.

Deaths

Between 2001 and 2008, the Consumer Product Safety Commission investigated 40 deaths associated with playground equipment. The average age of children who died was 6 years old. Of these, 27 (68%) died from strangulation and 6 (15%) died from falls to the playground surface. Most strangulation involved the combination of slides or swings and jump ropes, other ropes, dog leashes, or clothes drawstrings.

INJURY RISK FACTORS
All Emergency Department-Treated, Playground-Related Injuries

- While all children who use playgrounds are at risk for injury, boys sustain ED-treated injuries (55%) slightly more often than girls (45%).
- Children ages 5 to 9 have higher rates of ED visits for playground injuries than any other age group. Most of these injuries occur at school. On public playgrounds, more injuries occur on monkey bars and climbing equipment than on any other equipment.
- Playgrounds that are well maintained have fewer risks to children such as rusty or broken equipment.

Playground-Related Traumatic Brain Injury

- Boys more often sustain playground-related TBIs compared to girls.
- Most children who are treated for playground-related TBIs are 5 to 9 years of age.

- Playground-related TBIs varied by age group and equipment type:
- 0 to 4-year-olds are often injured on swings and slides.
- 5 to 9-year-olds are often injured on swings, monkey bars, and climbing equipment.
- 10 to 14-year-olds are often injured on swings, monkey bars, and climbing equipment.
- 5 to 14-year-olds sustain TBIs more frequently at school.

PUBLIC PLAYGROUND SAFETY CHECKLIST

Each year, more than 200,000 children go to U.S. hospital emergency rooms with injuries associated with playground equipment. Most injuries occur when a child falls from the equipment onto the ground.

Use this simple checklist to help make sure your local community or school playground is a safe place to play.

- Make sure surfaces around playground equipment have at least 12 inches of wood chips, mulch, sand, or pea gravel, or are mats made of safety-tested rubber or rubber-like materials.
- Check that protective surfacing extends at least 6 feet in all directions from play equipment. For swings, be sure surfacing extends, in back and front, twice the height of the suspending bar.
- Make sure play structures more than 30 inches high are spaced at least 9 feet apart.
- Check for dangerous hardware, like open "S" hooks or protruding bolt ends.
- Make sure spaces that could trap children, such as openings in guardrails or between ladder rungs, measure less than 3.5 inches or more than 9 inches.
- Check for sharp points or edges in equipment.
- Look out for tripping hazards, like exposed concrete footings, tree stumps, and rocks.
- Make sure elevated surfaces, like platforms and ramps, have guardrails to prevent falls.

- Check playgrounds regularly to see that equipment and surfacing are in good condition.
- Carefully supervise children on playgrounds to make sure they are safe.

Chapter 29 | **Sports Safety**

There are many ways to help reduce the risk of a concussion or other serious brain injury both on and off the sports field as follows.

CREATE A SAFE SPORT CULTURE[1]

Young athletes deserve to play sports in a culture that celebrates their hard work, dedication, and teamwork, and in programs that seek to create a safe environment—especially when it comes to concussion. As a youth sports coach or parent, your actions can create a safe sport culture and can lower an athlete's chance of getting a concussion or other serious injury.

Athletes thrive when they:

- Have fun playing their sport
- Receive positive messages and praise from their coaches for concussion symptom reporting
- Have parents who talk with them about concussion and model and expect safe play
- Get written instructions from a healthcare provider when to return to school and play
- Support their teammates sitting out of play if they have a concussion
- Feel comfortable reporting symptoms of a possible concussion to coaches

This chapter includes text excerpted from documents published by two public domain sources. Text under headings marked 1 are excerpted from "Brain Injury Safety Tips and Prevention," Centers for Disease Control and Prevention (CDC), February 27, 2020; Text under heading marked 2 is excerpted from "What Is a Concussion?" Centers for Disease Control and Prevention (CDC), February 12, 2019.

ENFORCE THE RULES[1]

Enforce the rules of the sport for fair play, safety, and sportsmanship. Ensure athletes avoid unsafe actions, such as:
- Striking another athlete on the head
- Using their head or helmet to contact another athlete
- Making illegal contacts or checking, tackling, or colliding with an unprotected opponent
- Trying to injure or put another athlete at risk for injury

Tell athletes you expect good sportsmanship at all times, both on and off the playing field.

WHAT IS CONCUSSION?[2]

A concussion is a type of traumatic brain injury (TBI) caused by a bump, blow, or jolt to the head or by a hit to the body that causes the head and brain to move rapidly back and forth. This sudden movement can cause the brain to bounce around or twist in the skull, creating chemical changes in the brain and sometimes stretching and damaging brain cells.

TALK ABOUT CONCUSSION REPORTING[1]

Talk with athletes about the importance of reporting a concussion.
Some athletes may not report a concussion because they do not think a concussion is serious. They may also worry about:
- Losing their position on the team or during the game
- Jeopardizing their future sports career
- Looking weak
- Letting their teammates down
- What their coach or teammates might think of them

GET A CONCUSSION ACTION PLAN IN PLACE[1]

Create an action plan that includes information on how to teach athletes ways to lower their chances of getting a concussion. If you think an athlete may have a concussion, you should:

- Remove the athlete from play.
- Keep an athlete with a possible concussion out of play on the same day of the injury and until cleared by a healthcare provider. Do not try to judge the severity of the injury yourself. Only a healthcare provider should assess an athlete for a possible concussion.
- Record and share information about the injury, such as how it happened and the athlete's symptoms, to help a healthcare provider assess the athlete.
- Inform the athlete's parent(s) or guardian(s) about the possible concussion and refer them to the Centers for Disease Control and Prevention's (CDC) website for concussion information.
- Ask for written instructions from the athlete's healthcare provider about the steps you should take to help the athlete safely return to play. Before returning to play an athlete should:
  - Be back to doing their regular school activities
  - Not have any symptoms from the injury when doing normal activities
  - Have the green-light from their healthcare provider to begin the return to play process

WHY THIS IS IMPORTANT[1]
Athletes May Try to Hide Concussion Symptoms.
- As many as 7 in 10 young athletes with a possible concussion report playing with concussion symptoms.
- Out of those, 4 in 10 said their coaches were unaware that they had a possible concussion.

Enforce Safe Play. You Set the Tone for Safety.
- As many as 25 percent of the concussions reported among high school athletes result from aggressive or illegal play.

Young Athletes Are More Likely to Play with a Concussion during a Big Game.

- In almost all sports, concussion rates are higher during competitions than in practice.
- Athletes may be less likely to tell their coach or athletic trainer about a possible concussion during a championship game or other important event.

Most Sports-Related Concussions Are Caused by Player-to-Player Contact.

- Over two-thirds (70%) of concussions among young athletes result from contact with another athlete.
- This is followed by player-to-surface contact (17%), such as hitting the ground or other obstacles.

Headache Is Most Commonly Reported Concussion Symptom.

- Almost all (94%) high school athletes with a concussion report having a headache.
- Other commonly reported symptoms include:
  - Dizziness (76%)
  - Trouble concentrating (55%)
  - Confusion (45%)
  - Bothered by light (36%)
  - Nausea (31%)

Chapter 30 | **Helmet Safety**

If you like recreational activities that involve wheels, concrete, or asphalt, then protect your brain by wearing a helmet.

Your helmet should fit properly and be:

- Well taken care of
- Age-appropriate
- Worn consistently and correctly
- Appropriately certified for use

While there is no concussion-proof helmet, a helmet can help protect you from a serious brain or head injury. Even with a helmet, it is important for you to avoid hits to the head.

FITTING YOUR HELMET

Your helmet should:

- Sit flat on your head—make sure it is level and is not tilted back or forward.
  - The front of the helmet should sit low—about two finger-widths above your eyebrows to protect your forehead.
- The straps on each side of your head should form a "Y" over your ears, with one part of the strap in front of your ear, and one behind—just below your earlobes.
  - If the helmet leans forward, adjust the rear straps. If it tilts backward, tighten the front straps.

This chapter contains text excerpted from the following sources: Text in this chapter begins with excerpts from "Helmet Safety," Centers for Disease Control and Prevention (CDC), August 28, 2018; Text under the heading "Frequently Asked Questions about Helmets" is excerpted from "Which Helmet for Which Activity?" U.S. Consumer Product Safety Commission (CPSC), May 16, 2014.

- Buckle the chinstrap securely at your throat so that the helmet feels snug on your head and does not wiggle up and down or from side to side.

HELMET MYTHS

- Many kids think helmets just are not cool. Who says helmets cannot be cool? If you are shopping for a helmet, there are lots of options, so you can pick out your favorite color. Or decorate your helmet with stickers and reflectors to show your personal style. Helmets are designed to help prevent injuries to your head. A serious fall or crash can cause permanent brain damage or death and that is definitely not cool.
- Today's helmets are lightweight, well ventilated, and have lots of padding. So, for those of you who think helmets just cannot be comfortable, try one on to make sure it fits properly and comfortably on your head before you buy it.
- Another myth about helmets is that a really good rider does not need to wear one. False! Bike crashes or collisions can happen at any time. Even professional bike racers get in serious wrecks. In three out of four bike crashes, bikers usually get some sort of injury to their head.

FREQUENTLY ASKED QUESTIONS ABOUT HELMETS
Why Are Helmets So Important?
For many recreational activities, wearing a helmet can reduce the risk of a severe head injury and even save your life.

How Does a Helmet Protect My Head?
During a typical fall or collision, much of the impact energy is absorbed by the helmet, rather than your head and brain.

Does This Mean That Helmets Prevent Concussions?
No. No helmet design has been proven to prevent concussions. The materials that are used in most of today's helmets are engineered

to absorb the high impact energies that can produce skull fractures and severe brain injuries. However, these materials have not been proven to counteract the energies believed to cause concussions. Beware of claims that a particular helmet can reduce or prevent concussions.

Are All Helmets the Same?

No. There are different helmets for different activities. Each type of helmet is made to protect your head from the kind of impacts that typically are associated with a particular activity or sport. Be sure to wear a helmet that is appropriate for the particular activity you are involved in. Helmets designed for other activities may not protect your head as effectively.

How Can I Tell Which Helmet Is the Right One to Use?

There are safety standards for most types of helmets. Bicycle and motorcycle helmets must comply with mandatory federal safety standards. Helmets for many other recreational activities are subject to voluntary safety standards.

Helmets that meet the requirements of a mandatory or voluntary safety standard are designed and tested to protect the user from receiving a skull fracture or severe brain injury while wearing the helmet. For example, all bicycle helmets manufactured after 1999 must meet the U.S. Consumer Product Safety Commission (CPSC) bicycle helmet standard (16 C.F.R. part 1203); helmets meeting this standard provide protection against skull fractures and severe brain injuries when the helmet is used properly.

The protection that the appropriate helmet can provide is dependent upon achieving a proper fit and wearing it correctly; for many activities, chin straps are specified in the standard, and they are essential for the helmet to function properly. For example, the bicycle standard requires that chin straps be strong enough to keep the helmet on the head and in the proper position during a fall or collision.

Helmets that meet a particular standard will contain a special label or marking that indicates compliance with that standard (usually found on the liner inside of the helmet, on the exterior surface, or attached to the chin strap). Do not rely solely on the helmet's name or appearance, or claims made on the packaging, to determine whether the helmet meets the appropriate requirements for your activity.

Do not choose style over safety. When choosing a helmet, avoid helmets that contain nonessential elements that protrude from the helmet (e.g., horns, Mohawks)—these may look interesting, but they may prevent the helmet's smooth surface from sliding after a fall, which could lead to injury.

Do not add anything to the helmet such as stickers, coverings, or other attachments that are not provided with the helmet, as such items can negatively affect the helmet's performance.

Avoid novelty and toy helmets that are made only to look like the real thing; such helmets are not made to comply with any standard and can be expected to offer little or no protection.

Are There Helmets That I Can Wear for More than One Activity?

Yes, but only a few. For example, you can wear a CPSC-compliant bicycle helmet while bicycling, recreational in-line skating or roller skating, or riding a kick scooter.

Are There Any Activities for Which One Should Not Wear a Helmet?

Yes. Children should not wear a helmet when playing on playgrounds or climbing trees. If a child wears a helmet during these activities, the helmet's chin strap can get caught on the equipment or tree branches and pose a risk of strangulation. The helmet may also prevent a child's head from moving through an opening that the body can fit through, and entrap the child by her or his head.

How Can I Tell If My Helmet Fits Properly?

A helmet should be both comfortable and snug. Be sure that the helmet is worn so that it is level on your head—not tilted back on the top of your head or pulled too low over your forehead. Once on your head, the helmet should not move in any direction, back-to-front or side-to-side. For helmets with a chin strap, be sure the chin strap is securely fastened so that the helmet does not move or fall off during a fall or collision.

If you buy a helmet for a child, bring the child with you so that the helmet can be tested for a good fit. Carefully examine the helmet and the accompanying instructions and safety literature.

What Can I Do If I Have Trouble Fitting the Helmet?

Depending on the type of helmet, you may have to apply the foam padding that comes with the helmet, adjust the straps, adjust the air bladders, or make other adjustments specified by the manufacturer. If these adjustments do not work, consult with the store where you bought the helmet or with the helmet manufacturer. Do not add extra padding or parts, or make any adjustments that are not specifically outlined in the manufacturer's instructions. Do not wear a helmet that does not fit correctly.

Will I Need to Replace a Helmet after an Impact?

That depends on the severity of the impact and whether the helmet was designed to withstand one impact (a single-impact helmet) or more than one impact (a multiple-impact helmet). For example, bicycle helmets are designed to protect against the impact of just a single fall, such as a bicyclist's fall onto the pavement. The foam material in the helmet will crush to absorb the impact energy during a fall or collision. The materials will not protect you again from an additional impact. Even if there are no visible signs of damage to the helmet, you must replace it after such an event.

Other helmets are designed to protect against multiple impacts. Two examples are football and ice hockey helmets. These helmets are designed to withstand multiple impacts of the type associated with the respective activities. However, you may still have to replace the helmet after one severe impact if the helmet has visible signs of damage, such as a cracked shell or permanent dent in the shell or liner. Consult the manufacturer's instructions or certification stickers on the helmet for guidance on when the helmet should be replaced.

How Long Are Helmets Supposed to Last?

Follow the guidance provided by the manufacturer. In the absence of such guidance, it may be prudent to replace your helmet within 5 to 10 years of purchase, a decision that can be based, at least in part, on how much the helmet was used, how it was cared for, and where it was stored. Cracks in the shell or liner, a loose shell, marks on the liner, fading of the shell, evidence of crushed foam in the liner, worn straps, and missing pads or other parts, are all reasons to replace a helmet. The regular replacement may minimize any reduced effectiveness that could result from the degradation of materials over time, and allow you to take advantage of recent advances in helmet protection.

Part 6 | Living with Traumatic Brain Injury

Chapter 31 | **Rehabilitation and Life after Traumatic Brain Injury**

REHABILITATION[1]

After experiencing a moderate or severe traumatic brain injury (TBI), people may need to be in a hospital until their medical condition improves. Some people need additional care after they leave the hospital, due to the effects of the TBI. Rehabilitation services can help people to restore or improve their ability to manage their lives and healthcare; stay involved with family, friends, and community, live at home, carry out daily activities, and find a job.

There are many choices for rehabilitation. People can receive these services at home, in hospitals, rehabilitation centers, day programs, supported living programs, or other places. People with TBI, their families, and their medical teams should work together with their health insurers to identify the best rehabilitation setting.

Trained rehabilitation professionals can test a person's abilities related to cognition, communication, language, behavior, movement, and management of their lives to develop a rehabilitation plan. Rehabilitation programs can involve many specialists, depending on the type of help a person needs. The rehabilitation plans can involve physical therapy, occupational therapy, speech and language therapy, physiatry (physical medicine), nursing,

This chapter includes text excerpted from documents published by two public domain sources. Text under headings marked 1 are excerpted from "Brain Injuries: Prevention, Rehabilitation, and Community Living," Administration for Community Living (ACL), June 18, 2015. Reviewed May 2020; Text under headings marked 2 are excerpted from "Report to Congress—Traumatic Brain Injury In the United States: Epidemiology and Rehabilitation," Centers for Disease Control and Prevention (CDC), June 15, 2013. Reviewed May 2020.

psychology, psychiatry, and social support. Initial treatment plans are frequently modified in response to a person's progress.

Rehabilitation can also identify ways to help people carry out tasks and daily activities. For example, a person may need reminders and timers to help with taking medicine or eating. Labels may be used to aid in remembering where food, clothes, dishes, and other things are. Written reminders can be used to organize days and help with how to prepare food, shop, and do other activities. For example, a person may not remember how to make a sandwich, or when to make or eat the sandwich.

EFFECTIVENESS OF TRAUMATIC BRAIN INJURY REHABILITATION[2]

Following hospitalization for a traumatic brain injury (TBI), people can receive rehabilitation care and services in various settings. Postacute rehabilitation is provided following an inpatient hospital stay and is typically indicated for people whose medical condition requires continued skilled nursing care. Some settings in which this level of rehabilitation is available includes inpatient rehabilitation facilities, longterm care hospitals, and skilled nursing facilities. people who no longer require skilled nursing care are usually discharged home and may receive rehabilitation care provided by outpatient and community service centers.

However, the type of rehabilitation care or setting selected is also based on a person's level of functional recovery, independence, geographic availability, and financial resources—including insurance coverage. For people living with TBI-related health effects, rehabilitation goals are structured to improve their independence in activities of daily living, social functioning, quality of life (QOL), and ability to participate in the community. They typically focus on the recovery of motor function, cognitive function, self-care skills, and community participation. A person's preinjury functioning and personal goals are fundamental in determining the best rehabilitation treatment plan, as well as the eventual outcomes. No single TBI rehabilitation program will work for all patients; rather, the goals and methods of rehabilitation must be individualized to each person.

TBI rehabilitation consists of therapies broadly categorized as cognitive and physical. Cognitive rehabilitation (CR) consists of a group of therapies used to manage deficits in thought processes and behavior (e.g., comprehension, perception, and learning). Physical rehabilitation focuses on enhancing different forms of mobility by improving physical factors, such as strength and endurance, as well as providing assistive devices that facilitate independence.

COGNITIVE REHABILITATION[2]

The Cognitive Rehabilitation (CR) Task Force of the American Congress of Rehabilitation Medicine (ACRM) Brain Injury-Interdisciplinary Special Interest Group (BI-ISIG) evaluated 370 studies and found that CR is effective during the postacute period—even 1 year or more after injury. Further analysis of the scientific literature suggests that CR is effective in patients with moderate and severe TBI. However, an Institute of Medicine (IOM) committee concluded that the evidence was insufficient to provide practice guidelines, particularly with respect to selecting the most effective treatments for a specific person. The insufficiency of the evidence was largely attributed to limitations in research designs for rehabilitation evaluation studies. And yet, empirical support for CR is growing with the strongest level of evidence for the following interventions:

- Direct attention training accompanied by metacognitive training to promote development of compensatory strategies and generalization
- Interventions to address functional communication deficits and memory strategies for mild memory impairments
- Meta-cognitive strategies for executive function deficits
- Comprehensive holistic neuropsychological rehabilitation

Preliminary evidence supports the effectiveness of group-based rehabilitation treatment of pragmatic communication disorders. However, research that demonstrates the effectiveness of cognitively based treatments for listening, speaking, reading, and writing, in social, educational, occupational, and community settings is lacking.

PHYSICAL REHABILITATION[2]

Evidence supports the general effectiveness of physical rehabilitation. With respect to specific interventions, regularly scheduled passive range-of-motion exercises and body repositioning are techniques that are commonly used with positive effects. Equipment, such as standing frames or tilt tables, can be used to maintain bone structure, elongate shortened muscles, challenge endurance, and stimulate the minimally conscious person. Bodyweight-supported (BWS) gait devices and knee-ankle-foot orthotics can be used with manual assistance to initiate standing postures. BWS devices can lead to improved cardiovascular function and assist with the beginning of walking training.

Gaming and virtual reality-based treatment methods are emerging as an adjunct to physical therapy standards of practice for treating people with TBI. One study demonstrated the effectiveness of improved goal-oriented, task-specific training with the use of a gaming system to promote practice of short sitting balance control for people with TBI. Another method used a game-based training tool that yielded an increase in practice volume and attention span, and furthermore, improvements in dynamic sitting balance control. Certain evidence indicates that virtual reality and other methods to improve vestibular function and balance result in improvements in both gait and gaze stability of people with TBI sustained during blasts. However, approaches such as motor interventions, proprioceptive muscle training, and neurodevelopmental treatment have been used in clinical practice with limited research on their effect on functional outcomes.

LIVING WITH A TRAUMATIC BRAIN INJURY[1]

People who experience TBIs that result in long-term health effects or disabilities can live productive, quality lives in their communities. Some government programs can help people and their families with health and long-term services and support. Medicare (www.

medicare.gov) generally covers health and rehabilitation for older adults and adults with disabilities who cannot work. Medicaid (www.medicaid.gov) generally covers health and rehabilitation services, plus help with daily activities for those who qualify—primary people of all ages with low incomes and limited assets. Since states control who gets Medicaid services and the type and amount of services available, programs vary across the country. The Administration for Community Living (ACL) (www.acl.gov) has information about services and supports for people who experience disability. The U.S. Veterans Health Administration (VHA) (www.va.gov/health) can provide certain health and long-term services and support to qualified veterans with TBI. In addition, many groups are doing research that may help people with TBIs and their families.

Someone who has a disability due to aging or a disease or injury other than TBI may also have a TBI. A study of adults in one state found that almost 40 percent of community-living adults who reported having a disability also reported that they had had at least one TBI with loss of consciousness sometime in their life.

There is growing evidence that a TBI is not just an isolated event; instead, a person's brain can continue to change years after a moderate or severe TBI. Some people continue to improve, while others may get worse. Few stay the same. Healthy brain habits are good for everyone, but especially smart for someone who has already experienced a TBI. Meet regularly with your healthcare team, and take care of your health. For example:

- Eat a healthy diet that is low in salt, solid fats, and simple sugars.
- Avoid drinking alcohol.
- Get active and stay active every day.
- Find time every day to relax and meditate.
- Sleep seven to eight hours each night.
- Learn new things every day.
- Connect with your family, friends, and communities.

Chapter 32 | **Traumatic Brain Injuries and Further Injuries**

Prevent traumatic brain injuries (TBIs) and future unintentional injuries by understanding the risks. Brain injury awareness month is an important time to highlight the lifelong effects of a TBI. A TBI is caused by a bump, blow, or jolt to the head, or a penetrating head injury that disrupts the normal function of the brain. People who have had a moderate-to-severe TBI may experience changes in thinking and balance, which may put them at greater risk of later unintentional injuries. TBIs also increase the risk of dying from several other causes. For example, compared to people without TBI, people with TBI are more likely to die from:
- Seizures: 50 times more likely
- Unintentional drug poisoning: 11 times more likely
- Infections: 9 times more likely
- Pneumonia: 6 times more likely

The leading causes of TBIs include falls among older adults, being struck by or against an object, assaults, and motor vehicle crashes. Current efforts to reduce unintentional injuries include preventing older adult falls, improving sports concussion culture, and increasing motor vehicle safety. This public-health approach to injury prevention can reduce the rate of TBI and its long-term consequences.

This chapter includes text excerpted from "TBIs and Injuries," Centers for Disease Control and Prevention (CDC), March 21, 2017.

PREVENTING OLDER ADULT FALLS

According to the Centers for Disease Control and Prevention (CDC) data, almost 8 in 10 TBIs among older adults are caused by a fall. Emergency department (ED) visits more than doubled from 2007–2013, reaching more than 394,000 visits. Hospitalizations increased by almost 50 percent, resulting in more than 91,000 stays. Falls are preventable. Here are some steps that older adults can take to prevent falls:

- Talk to your doctor.
- Do strength and balance exercises.
- Have your eyes checked.
- Make your home safe.

IMPROVING SPORTS CONCUSSION CULTURE

The CDC has a new educational gaming app designed to teach children six to eight years of age about basic concussion safety. Children can learn the benefits of playing it safe and smart through a futuristic world of galactic racing adventures. The app teaches children about the different ways the brain can get hurt during sports activities and how important it is to tell a coach, parent, or other adults when an injury occurs.

Based on the CDC's research, it is known that prevention is possible. The CDC has have made youth sports concussion one of their focus areas, but they cannot solve this issue alone. All of us play a role in creating a culture of concussion safety. Here is how:

- Change the "win-at-all costs" mentality.
- Talk to your athletes about concussion.
- Model, expect, and reinforce safe play.
- Get concussion information on every sideline.

INCREASING MOTOR VEHICLE SAFETY

For youth and young adults, motor vehicle crashes were the main cause of TBI-related deaths and accounted for 56 percent of TBI-related deaths among 5 to 14 year-olds, and 47 percent of TBI-related deaths for 15 to 24 year-olds from 2006–2010. Everyone can improve motor vehicle safety by:

- Using seat belts on every trip, no matter how short. Make sure passengers buckle up too.
- Buckling children in age and size-appropriate car seats, booster seats, and seat belts. Those 12 years of age and under should be buckled in the back seat.
- Choosing not to drive after drinking alcohol or using drugs and helping others do the same
- Knowing your state's graduated driver licensing laws, and consider using tools, such as the CDC's parent-teen driving agreement if you are the parent of a teen driver

Chapter 33 | **Managing Specific Traumatic Brain Injury Symptoms**

POOR CONCENTRATION

The main cause of poor concentration is tiredness. When it becomes difficult to concentrate on what you are doing, take a break and relax. Between 15 and 30 minutes a day should be enough. If you still continue to have problems, your work day, class schedule, or daily routine should be temporarily shortened. Trying to stick to it will not help, and usually makes things worse.

Reducing distractions can help. Turn down the radio or try to work where it is quiet. At first, avoiding noisy environments may be helpful, then return to them gradually. Do not try to do too many things at once. Writing while you talk on the phone or taking notes as you listen to someone are examples of doing two things at the same time. It may be difficult for you to concentrate on more than one thing at first. You will be better able to concentrate when you have had enough rest. So, if you really need to concentrate on something important, do so when you are feeling fresh.

FATIGUE

It is normal to be more tired after a head injury. Most people experience some degree of fatigue during their recovery. The only sensible treatment for being tired is rest. Avoid wearing yourself out.

This chapter includes text excerpted from "Traumatic Brain Injury: A Guide for Patients," U.S. Department of Veterans Affairs (VA), January 18, 2009. Reviewed May 2020.

Gradually increase your activity level. You may find that you need to sleep more than usual, in which case it is a good idea to get the extra sleep that you need. Most patients have more energy in the morning than later in the day. An afternoon nap can help if you find that it is harder to do things at the end of the day. Physical and mental fatigue usually diminishes over time; it should be greatly improved within six months after a brain injury.

It may seem counterintuitive, but a well-designed exercise program can help your physical and mental endurance. Adding activity gradually is the key. For instance, an hour of morning activity may be all that you can handle. From there, you slowly and incrementally add activity followed by rest breaks. Closely monitor your fatigue levels until you reach an acceptable level that you can tolerate, and be careful to avoid extreme fatigue.

Simple suggestions to reduce fatigue:
- Follow a regular sleep schedule and reduce disruptions. Try to sleep for at least eight hours per night.
- Take scheduled naps and rest breaks, but be increasingly active in between.
- Do strenuous activities when energy is normally highest and rest when energy is normally lowest.
- Simplify tasks whenever possible—conserve your energy.
- Add tasks only as you can tolerate them, slowly and incrementally.
- Set a cut-off time for ending daily activities.
- Plan proper nutrition. Eat healthier foods and stay on a fairly structured routine.
- Use stress management and relaxation techniques.
- Get help to become and stay organized.
- Start a diary to understand patterns and triggers of fatigue.

SLEEP DIFFICULTIES

You might expect that the fatigue you experience during recovery would cause you to sleep more soundly. However, sleep disturbance is actually quite common following a brain injury. Studies have shown that individuals who suffer a brain injury often have difficulty getting to sleep and maintaining uninterrupted sleep at night, and thus experience excessive daytime sleepiness. When they do sleep, their sleep is lighter and less restful, and they frequently awaken. Getting adequate sleep is very important in the healing process. If you do not sleep well at night, you will be more tired during the day. When you are tired during the day, you will find it difficult to concentrate, and may become irritable and angry more easily. Thus, lack of sleep can exacerbate your other symptoms.

Simple suggestions to improve your sleep habits and routines:

- Wake up at roughly the same time each morning.
- Avoid caffeine, especially in the evenings.
- Avoid exercising late in the evening.
- Set your bedroom temperature to a comfortable level.
- Ensure that your bedroom is quiet and dark.
- If you take daytime naps, try to rest long enough to re-energize (30 minutes or less should be sufficient), but not so long that you will have difficulty falling asleep in the evening.

IRRITABILITY AND EMOTIONAL CHANGES

Some people show emotions more easily after a brain injury. They may yell at people or say things they would not normally say, or get annoyed easily by things that normally would not upset them. Some may even get violent. You may also find that you get more emotional in other ways, getting frustrated or tearful when you normally would not. This behavior does not necessarily mean that you are feeling a deep emotion, but can occur because the brain is not regulating emotions to the same extent as before the injury. If any of these episodes happen, it is usually a sign that it is time to take a rest from what you are doing and get away from it. There are a variety of different techniques to deal with irritability. Some people find that leaving the frustrating situation temporarily is helpful. Others employ relaxation techniques or attempt to use up emotional energy through exercise. One frequent cause of irritability and emotionality is fatigue. People lose their tempers more easily when they are tired or overworked. Adjust your schedule and get more rest if you notice yourself becoming irritable or emotional.

Everyone gets angry from time to time, often with good reason. Being irritable only becomes a problem when it interferes with your ability to get along with people from day to day. If you find yourself getting into arguments that cause trouble at home or work, try to change the way you think about things. Thoughts often make us more angry than what actually happened. You can see this yourself by imagining an irritating situation and why it would make you angry.

There is usually a reason that irritating things happen. When something makes you angry, ask yourself what caused it. Family, friends, or co-workers can do things that bother us at times. Try to think of why they did whatever it was that irritated you. What would they say the reason was? Thinking about what caused a problem is the first step toward solving it.

Problems can usually be solved better if you stay calm and explain your point of view. The steps you need to take to solve a problem will be the same when you are calm as they would be if you were irritated. Try to remind yourself of this when you find yourself becoming irritable.

You can usually come up with several ways to solve a problem. Try to think of at least five different ways, and then decide on which is best. Just realizing that there are several things you can do to solve a problem will make it a lot less irritating.

DEPRESSION

For reasons we do not fully understand, depression seems to occur more often after a brain injury. More than one-third of people with recent traumatic brain injury (TBI) become depressed, especially during the first year after injury. One reason for this increase in depression may be because brain injury causes an imbalance in certain chemicals in the brain and disrupts brain networks critical for mood regulation.

Another cause of depression in TBI may be psychological and social changes such as losing friends, losing abilities, and not being able to return to work or other meaningful activities after injury.

Simply put, people become depressed when unpleasant things happen to them, and a head injury is unpleasant. We feel good when good things happen to us. Thus, an effective way to treat depression is to make sure that good things happen. One way to do this is to plan to do something enjoyable for yourself each day. Make your plan specific, and then be sure to stick to it. Decide on an activity you like and exactly when you are going to do it. That way you can look forward to it. Anticipating and doing enjoyable things each day will improve your mood.

Chances are that if you are depressed, you are telling yourself things that are depressing. Thinking that the situation is terrible, that there is no end to it in sight, that you are not able to do anything about it, and that it is your fault are all depressing things to tell yourself. Thinking this way can become a habit if you do it enough. Usually, when people tell themselves unpleasant things all the time it is out of habit, not because those things are really true. If you find yourself thinking depressing thoughts, stop. Simply stopping a depressing thought can make you feel better. See if what you are telling yourself is really true.

MEMORY PROBLEMS

Memory difficulties have several causes. The part of our brain that stores memories is called the "temporal lobe." This is the part of the brain that is most likely to be bruised in a head injury. Some memory difficulties can be caused by the bruises, which is why you may not remember the accident very well. Like a black and blue mark on your arm or leg, these bruises will recover with time. Your memory will most likely improve as this happens. Most of the memory problems that patients notice after a head injury are not caused by bruising. They usually come from poor concentration and being tired. For you to remember something, you have to pay attention to it first. If you do not concentrate long enough, the information is never stored in your memory. Concentration problems are a normal part of recovering from a head injury and some memory trouble is a normal side effect of this. You will probably be able to concentrate and remember better when you get enough rest. Memory problems can be a sign that you are pushing

Table 33.1. Things We Normally Forget

"Symptom"	Percentage
Forgets telephone numbers	58 percent
Forgets people's names	48 percent
Forgets where car was parked	32 percent
Loses car keys	31 percent
Forgets groceries	28 percent
Forgets reason for entering room	27 percent
Forgets directions	24 percent
Forgets appointment dates	20 percent
Forgets store locations in mall	20 percent
Loses items around the house	17 percent
Loses wallet or pocketbook	17 percent
Forgets content of daily conversations	17 percent

yourself too hard. Writing important things down, using a pocket tape recorder, and asking for reminders are other excellent ways of coping with temporary memory difficulties. They will help recovery and not slow it down.

Of course, nobody's memory is perfect anyway. After a head injury, it can be easy to forget that we sometimes had trouble remembering things even before the accident. Some of the symptoms you notice may actually have nothing to do with your head injury. A list of common memory problems is shown below along with the percentage of people who experience each symptom even though they did not have a head injury.

Worrying about remembering things that you would normally forget can make your memory seem worse to you. If you can remember your memory problems, you probably do not have much of a memory problem! People with serious memory difficulties are usually not upset by their symptoms. They do not remember that they have any memory trouble.

HEADACHES

Headaches are part of the normal recovery process, but that does not make them any less bothersome. Not only are they painful to experience, but frequent headaches can take a toll on you mentally and emotionally, and are a common cause of irritability and concentration problems following a head injury. This guide cannot replace the medical advice that you should get if you are bothered by headaches. Headaches can have many causes, and your doctor will want to diagnose the problem and prescribe medication that can help if you need it.

One of the most common causes of headaches after a head injury is stress or tension. This is usually the cause when the headaches start for the first time several weeks after the injury. These headaches mean that you are trying to do too much. They will probably disappear if you take a break and relax. Your workday, class schedule, or daily routine should be temporarily shortened if you continue to have headaches. Stress or worry cause tension headaches by increasing muscle tension in your neck or forehead. These muscles become tense and can stay tight without you realizing it, out of habit. They can become even tighter once a headache starts, because muscles automatically tense in reaction to pain. This muscle tension makes the headaches worse.

If you have tension headaches, relaxing your muscles can help. One way to do this is with a method called "progressive muscle relaxation." Start by clenching your hand into a fist, as hard as you can. Notice how the muscle tension feels. Now relax your hand completely and notice the difference. Now clench both your hands as hard as you can and hold them that way for a moment or two before letting them relax completely. Notice the difference. Now continue to tense and relax more muscle groups by adding a different set each time: hands, arms, face, chest, stomach, buttocks, legs, feet. This method works best if you are lying on your back. Finally, tense all the muscles in your body at once as hard as you can, and then let them relax. At this point all your muscles will be very relaxed. Progressive muscle relaxation can help prevent tension headaches by relaxing your muscles. This works best if you practice it each day at about the same time for five minutes or so. But, be sure that you do not use this technique while you are having a headache.

ANXIETY

Worry about symptoms and problems at work is the main cause of anxiety for many patients. Anxiety should not be a problem for you if you understand that your symptoms are a normal part of recovery, get enough rest, and gradually increase your responsibilities at work. If you are anxious, chances are that you are telling yourself things that are making you that way. Usually, when people worry all the time it is out of habit, not because the things that they are telling themselves are really true. The steps you need to take to solve a problem will be the same when you are calm as they would be if you were anxious. If you find yourself thinking anxious thoughts, stop. Simply stopping an anxious thought can make you feel better. See if what you are telling yourself is really true.

CONFUSION AND TROUBLE THINKING

Many people feel uncertain, perplexed, or confused after a head injury. They find that their mind and feelings do not react in the ways they used to. They may fear that they are going crazy. This is a normal reaction to a head injury. If you have these feelings, it is good to talk about them with someone you trust.

Trouble thinking is often a side effect of other symptoms. Concentration problems, being tired, headaches, and anxiety can all make it hard to think clearly. Like these other symptoms, trouble thinking is probably a sign that you are doing too much too soon.

DIZZINESS, VISUAL DIFFICULTIES, AND LIGHT SENSITIVITY

Dizziness and visual difficulties should be checked by your doctor. These symptoms usually go away by themselves in three to six months or less in most patients. If you find these symptoms troublesome, your doctor may want to prescribe medication for motion sickness, or eyeglasses. Some motion sickness medications are very effective for dizziness, but can make you drowsy or reduce your attention span as side effects.

You may notice some increased sensitivity to bright light or loud noise, particularly if you have headaches. Some increased sensitivity is normal after a head injury. But, scientific studies by neurosurgeons and neuropsychologists in New Zealand show that a person's actual sensitivity to light and noise has nothing to do with how much light and noise bother them. Paying attention to these symptoms makes them seem worse, because paying attention to a feeling seems to magnify or increase it. The less you think and worry about your symptoms, the faster they will usually go away.

Chapter 34 | Traumatic Brain Injuries and the Role of Parents

HOW CAN I HELP KEEP MY CHILDREN OR TEENS SAFE?

Sports are a great way for children and teens to stay healthy and help them do well in school. To help lower your children's or teens' chances of getting a concussion or other serious brain injury, you should:

- Help create a culture of safety for the team.
- Work with their coach to teach ways to lower the chances of getting a concussion.
- Emphasize the importance of reporting concussions and taking time to recover from one.
- Ensure that they follow their coach's rules for safety and the rules of the sport.
- Tell your children or teens that you expect them to practice good sportsmanship at all times.
- When appropriate for the sport or activity, teach your children or teens that they must wear a helmet to lower the chances of the most serious types of brain or head injury. There is no "concussion-proof" helmet. Even with a helmet, it is important for children and teens to avoid hits to the head.

This chapter includes text excerpted from "A Fact Sheet for Youth Sports Parents," Centers for Disease Control and Prevention (CDC), August 2019.

HOW CAN I SPOT A POSSIBLE CONCUSSION?

Children and teens who show or report one or more of the signs and symptoms listed below—or simply say they just "don't feel right" after a bump, blow, or jolt to the head or body—may have a concussion or other serious brain injury.

Signs Observed by Parents

- Appears dazed or stunned
- Forgets an instruction, is confused about an assignment or position, or is unsure of the game, score, or opponent
- Moves clumsily
- Answers questions slowly
- Loses consciousness (even briefly)
- Shows mood, behavior, or personality changes
- Cannot recall events prior to or after a hit or fall

Symptoms Reported by Children and Teens

- Headache or "pressure" in head
- Nausea or vomiting
- Balance problems or dizziness, or double or blurry vision
- Bothered by light or noise
- Feeling sluggish, hazy, foggy, or groggy
- Confusion, or concentration or memory problems
- Just not "feeling right," or "feeling down"

While most children and teens with a concussion feel better within a couple of weeks, some will have symptoms for months or longer. Talk with your children's or teens' healthcare provider if their concussion symptoms do not go away or if they get worse after they return to their regular activities.

WHAT ARE SOME MORE SERIOUS DANGER SIGNS TO LOOK OUT FOR?

In rare cases, a dangerous collection of blood (hematoma) may form on the brain after a bump, blow, or jolt to the head or body and can squeeze the brain against the skull. Call 911, or take your child or teen to the emergency department right away if, after a bump, blow, or jolt to the head or body, she or he has one or more of these danger signs:

- One pupil larger than the other
- Drowsiness or inability to wake up
- A headache that gets worse and does not go away
- Slurred speech, weakness, numbness, or decreased coordination
- Repeated vomiting or nausea, convulsions or seizures (shaking or twitching)
- Unusual behavior, increased confusion, restlessness, or agitation
- Loss of consciousness (passed out/knocked out). Even a brief loss of consciousness should be taken seriously.

Chapter 35 | **Supporting Brain Development in Traumatized Children and Youth**

Healthy brain development is essential for realizing one's full potential and for overall well being. For children and youth who experience child abuse or neglect and associated trauma, brain development may be interrupted, leading to functional impairments. Ongoing maltreatment can alter a child's brain development and affect mental, emotional, and behavioral health into adulthood. Frontline child welfare professionals are in a unique position to recognize developmental delays in children and youth and provide appropriate support services. This chapter summarizes what you can do to promote healthy brain development for this vulnerable group of children and youth and put families and service providers in touch with the most effective, evidence-based interventions.

UNDERSTANDING TRAUMA AND BRAIN DEVELOPMENT

Early life experiences shape the development of brain circuitry and help to determine the makeup of a person's intelligence, emotions, and personality. Positive experiences with caregivers, family

This chapter includes text excerpted from "Supporting Brain Development in Traumatized Children and Youth," Child Welfare Information Gateway, U.S. Department of Health and Human Services (HHS), September 2017.

members, and the broader community strongly influence whether an infant or child develops a strong or weak foundation for future social-emotional health and help the child's developing brain offset the potentially negative consequences of abuse or neglect.

When infants and young children are exposed to chronic or acute maltreatment within the caregiving context, brain development may be compromised and emotional, behavioral, or learning challenges may persist, especially in the absence of targeted and trauma-informed interventions.

When primary caregivers make infants and children feel safe and nurtured, their developing brains are able to spend more time learning and building essential connections. When children feel unsafe or threatened, however, their brains shift into survival mode, making learning particularly difficult.

Brain imaging studies of children with documented cases of maltreatment reveal distinct changes in both the brain's structure and functioning. Such studies show that abuse, neglect, and other exposure to trauma can result in long-lasting negative changes to the brain. Victims of child maltreatment frequently suffer from delayed speech, reading ability, and school readiness. Although these results could be related to other variables as well, the correlation between childhood abuse and neglect and altered brain functioning appears significant in brain imaging studies:

- The area of the brain associated with executive functioning and planning, the prefrontal cortex, shows correspondingly smaller amounts of gray and white matter in youth who were studied for their reported experiences with childhood trauma compared with those who did not report such experiences.
- The region of the brain associated with learning, the hippocampus region, is smaller in individuals reporting early exposure to trauma.
- The brain's emotional reaction center associated with behavioral functioning and survival instincts, the amygdala, shows correspondingly increased reactivity with higher reported exposure to trauma during infancy and early childhood.

Trauma-induced changes to the brain can result in varying degrees of cognitive impairment and emotional dysregulation that can lead to a host of problems, including difficulty with attention and focus, learning disabilities, low self-esteem, impaired social skills, and sleep disturbances. Since trauma exposure has been linked to a significantly increased risk of developing several mental and behavioral health issues—including posttraumatic stress disorder (PTSD), depression, anxiety, bipolar disorder, and substance use disorders—it is important for practitioners to be aware of steps they can take to help minimize the neurological effects of child abuse and neglect and promote healthy brain development.

ENCOURAGING HEALTHY BRAIN DEVELOPMENT

A child welfare professional can help support healthy brain development by promoting safe and nurturing environments for children and families and by encouraging both the prevention and treatment of trauma.

Preventing Trauma

Efforts to support healthy brain development ideally should start before and continue through pregnancy, when maternal health can influence the developing brain and the mother-child attachment begins. Maternal stress can affect the developing brain and create long term issues for the unborn child. Child welfare professionals can help parents and caregivers focus on optimal fetal, newborn, and child development by linking families to services designed for at-risk expectant families, such as home visiting programs. Home visiting programs teach caregivers specific parenting skills—techniques for coping with a baby's crying or other behavioral challenges, for example—and have been linked with reduced stress in the family environment.

Healthy brain development can be encouraged after birth through supportive services, such as continued home visits and other parent education programs. Information Gateway's website features extensive resources on protective factors that professionals can use to strengthen families and help prevent trauma, including the following:

- Nurturing and attachment
- Parental education regarding child and youth development
- Parental resilience
- Social connections
- Concrete supports for parents
- Social and emotional competence for children

Enhancing Caregiver Interactions and Building Relationships

Child welfare professionals can help parents and caregivers by talking with them about child development, including important developmental milestones, how each child has a different time-table for reaching those milestones, and how quality interaction with the child can enhance her or his development. Helping parents and caregivers increase their sensitivity and responsiveness to their child's needs can make a tremendous difference in that child's future mental health and well-being. Child welfare professionals can help ensure that a child has a positive, enduring relationship with at least one important person in her or his life. For instance, training relative caregivers or foster parents to meet the child's emotional and behavioral needs can help promote healthy bonds that support the child's development. If the child has been placed in out-of-home care, you can facilitate quality visits between the birth parent and the child. You can also ensure that the birth family, resource family, and any other caregivers are all receiving the same advice regarding parenting and attachment techniques.

The predictability of a routine gives a child the sense that the world is a safe place for exploring, learning, and growing. This is important to the developing brain because it lowers stress and reinforces a sense of wellbeing. Child welfare professionals can help parents and caregivers understand the importance of consistency for children and suggest an age-appropriate plan. A routine also allows caregivers to establish limits for challenging behavior and disciplinary strategies, which should be applied consistently and fairly. Consistency is very important to the developing infant and child, and caregivers should be very clear with children if, and when, there will be changes to routines.

To help strengthen the bond between caregiver and child and create safe environments for the families in your care, see Gateway's Parent Education to Strengthen Families and Reduce the Risk of Maltreatment at (www.childwelfare.gov/pubs/issue-briefs/parented/) and the Centers for Disease Control and Prevention (CDC) guide, Essentials for Childhood Framework: Steps to Create Safe, Stable, Nurturing Relationships and Environments for All Children, at (www.cdc.gov/ViolencePrevention/childmaltreatment/essentials/index. html). You can also consult the Triple P Positive Parenting Program, an evidence-based program shown to improve parent-child interactions, at (www.ct.gov/triplep/lib/triplep/pdfs/triplepoverview.pdf).

Supporting Brain Development in Older Children

Another critical phase of human brain development occurs during adolescence, offering youth the potential to recover from earlier trauma and set a new foundation for the years ahead. Positive experiences during this pivotal phase can strengthen healthy neural connections and promote learning. Child welfare staff, and others working with young people, can create opportunities to engage in trauma-informed practice and provide supports that may help reverse the harmful impacts of prior trauma. According to the Jim Casey Youth Opportunities Initiative (2011), child welfare professionals can do this in the following ways:

- Develop an understanding of trauma and its impact on child and youth development.
- Recognize that youth can be traumatized by systems and services designed to help them.
- Create safe and welcome spaces for young people.
- Share information about trauma, complex trauma, ambiguous loss, neuroplasticity, and resilience to increase their understanding of the developmental needs of older youth.

Trusted adults can provide a needed safety net at this vulnerable time and offer youth advice and support regarding their growing independence.

You can help the important adults in a preteen's life understand how the brain develops and educate them about strategies that will help youth with the following:

- Organizational and goal-setting skills
- Decision-making skills
- Stress management techniques
- Wellness practices (e.g., balanced diet, ample sleep, avoidance of risky behaviors)

SCREENING CHILDREN FOR SERVICES AND WORKING WITH OTHER PROVIDERS

It is important for children who have experienced trauma to receive screening as soon as possible to check for potential developmental delays. Determining whether the children and youth in your care require services can make a substantial difference in their future health and well-being, as early treatment may prevent additional developmental delays or deficits and increase the likelihood of favorable outcomes.

The CDC lists the following as risk factors for developmental delays (U.S. Department of Health and Human Services (HHS), 2015):

- Medical factors such as low birthweight, premature or multiples birth, or brain damage experienced in utero or later
- Genetic factors or maternal or paternal mental-health issues
- Unhealthy parental behaviors during pregnancy, such as drinking or smoking
- Exposure of mother or child to high levels of environmental toxins

Collaborating with multiple providers across varied service sectors may help improve outcomes for children and youth since no single system can address all the issues a child and family may experience.

Early Intervention

Each State has an early intervention program (EIP) that provides specialized health, education, and therapeutic services to infants and toddlers who have an identified developmental delay or disability. EIPs can support families in addressing children's developmental delays through parenting training, home visitations, respite care, or other supports. When a family is referred to an EIP, the EIP service coordinator will work with the family to develop an individual family service plan and coordinate with the child welfare system to make sure the child's needs are being met. According to the Early Childhood Technical Assistance Center (ECTAC), early intervention services result in greater developmental progress for between 67 percent and 75 percent of participating children across three outcomes—social relationships, the use of knowledge and skills, and taking action to meet needs—and most children receiving such services leave the program functioning within age-level expectations (ECTAC, 2016).

Quality Early Care and Education

Early care and education (ECE) professionals can be critical partners in supporting healthy brain development and in helping to overcome the effects of an unhealthy home environment. Young children often spend a substantial amount of time in ECE settings, and ECE professionals may be among the first to observe signs of developmental delays. ECE programs that encourage regular communication with families can help professionals to flag developmental concerns, connect families to needed services, reduce stress, and improve outcomes (The National Scientific Council on the Developing Child, 2013). Children's stress responses have been shown to return to normal through relationships with supportive and responsive caregivers and high-quality early education services.

Many States have instituted a quality rating system for ECE. The National Association for the Education of Young Children (NAEYC) has set 10 standards for early childhood programs. To earn accreditation, programs must meet all 10 standards.

Schools and Communities

Children whose brain development has been compromised by trauma may face significant problems in their schools and communities, including absenteeism, poor academic performance, and behavioral issues. These problems are often compounded when children fall behind their peers in school and have difficulty making and maintaining social connections. You can reach out to school staff regarding the children you serve to inform them of each child's individual needs and to seek accommodations to ensure their educational success. School officials may benefit in particular from special training on the impact of trauma and from guidance on how to work with traumatized children and youth.

The National Child Traumatic Stress Network (NCTSN) has developed tools and materials to help educators understand and respond to the specific needs of traumatized children.

Mental Health

Children and youth affected neurologically by trauma may experience a variety of emotional regulation and/ or behavioral challenges that require attention by a mental-health professional. An assessment by a trained professional can help determine if the child or youth would be best served by individual or group therapy and which type of therapy would be most appropriate. When parental or primary caregiver stress and unresolved trauma from the parent's childhood are a factor in parent (or caregiver) and child well-being, treatment may be necessary for both children and guardians.

TREATMENT FOR TRAUMA-AFFECTED CHILDREN AND YOUTH

There are several promising evidence-based intervention models for helping to restore social, emotional, and cognitive health in infants, children, and youth who have experienced developmental deficits from traumatic stress. These treatments aim to reduce the harmful effects of toxic stress by restoring the balance between the emotional and cognitive systems of the brain. Treatment may include teaching children how to self-calm and regulate emotions;

how to process their experience through images, thoughts, emotions, and movement to engage all parts of the brain and encourage positive emotions and initiative; and a family component to address communication patterns, conflict, and hierarchy. The type and length of intervention will depend on the degree of impairment and the services that are available in your area. The following are examples of interventions that can help support brain health.

Attachment and Biobehavioral Catchup

Attachment and biobehavioral catchup (ABC) interventions are designed for caregivers of infants and very young children up to 2 years of age who have suffered from neglect. ABC takes place in the caregiver's home and includes both the caregiver and affected child over a 10-session treatment sequence. The sessions are designed to instruct the caregiver on how to best nurture the child and how routine interactions can optimize the child's healthy development. Studies of ABC interventions have shown them to be successful in reducing a child's stress hormones, which improves a child's overall well-being.

Child–parent Psychotherapy

Child–parent psychotherapy (CPP) is a flexible two-way model targeted to young children from infancy through 6 years of age with attachment, behavioral, or mental-health problems from exposure to maltreatment, domestic violence, or other trauma. CPP can be used with birth parents, foster parents, or kinship parents and can also be adjusted for transitions among caregivers.

Therapy is designed to repair trust in the relationship between the child and primary caregiver through restoring the child's sense of safety and building the primary caregiver's sense of competence in parenting skills. CPP also considers current socioeconomic stressors and cultural values, such as those experienced in immigrant families, and it creates an opportunity for caregivers to understand their own emotions surrounding unresolved losses or traumas from earlier experiences. CPP is conducted in weekly sessions with the parent or primary caregiver and child over the course of a year.

Parent–Child Interaction Therapy

Parent–child interaction therapy (PCIT) is designed for children 2 to 12 years of age and is used to address interpersonal trauma and repair the caregiver–child relationship by building responsive parenting skills. PCIT takes place through the active coaching of primary caregivers during caregiver–child play sessions. Coaching takes place in real time behind a one-way mirror during a caregiver–child play session—with a hearing device in the caregiver's ear—so that coaching is concealed from the child. The goal of PCIT is to build responsive parenting skills and a secure parent–child relationship based on nurturing care, firm control, and effective communication where clear limit setting results in consistent discipline and positive behavior.

Eye Movement Desensitization and Reprocessing

Eye movement desensitization and reprocessing (EMDR) is a clinical psychotherapy technique used with all age groups—from very young children to adults—where the emotional or behavioral problems associated with past trauma exposure are alleviated by the active "reprocessing" of traumatic memories. This reprocessing allows the individual to establish a healthier frame of mind. The length of treatment will depend on many factors, including whether single-episode or chronic and complex trauma exposure is involved. In general, the treatment must progress through eight distinct phases that incorporate past memories, current triggers, and positive responses for the future.

Integrative Treatment of Complex Trauma

Integrative treatment of complex trauma (ITCT) is designed for children and youth who have experienced complex psychological trauma. These children frequently present with parental attachment issues (e.g., parental abandonment, multiple foster placements). ITCT employs multiple treatment modalities, including relational treatment in individual and group therapy, and cognitive exposure and play therapies. There are separate programs for children (ITCT-C for 8 to 12 years of age) and adolescents (ICTC-A for 13 to 21 years of age).

Trauma-Focused Cognitive Behavioral Therapy

Trauma-focused cognitive behavioral therapy (TF-CBT) is targeted to children 3 to 18 years of age and their families to address significant trauma-induced emotional or behavioral difficulties. At its core, CBT is based on the premise that individuals' thoughts, perceptions, and attitudes about themselves and others affect their interpretation of external events and related emotions and behaviors. CBT seeks to inform individuals' awareness of their cognitive distortions and the behavior patterns that reinforce such thinking. TF-CBT is a structured child and parent model that combines elements of cognitive therapy, behavioral therapy, and family therapy to eliminate a child's negative emotional and behavioral responses to trauma and provides primary caregivers with the tools to address the child's emotional distress. When possible, TF-CBT is conducted with children and primary caregivers in separate, parallel sessions.

Trauma Systems Therapy

Trauma systems therapy (TST) is both a clinical and an organizational model designed for children and youth 6 through 19 years of age affected by trauma to coordinate a broad-based approach to trauma care. TST enlists the family, neighborhood, school, and community in meeting a child's needs and recognizing her or his strengths and weaknesses. It relies on a two-pronged approach that builds the child's capacity to self-regulate powerful emotions and equips the child's social environment to help the child manage these emotions and protect against threats.

Mindfulness Meditation

Mindfulness meditation has shown promise for improving mental, behavioral, and physical outcomes in youth who have experienced trauma. Mindfulness therapy is similar to CBT and involves retraining an individual's attention on the present moment. Brain imaging studies with combat veterans demonstrate that mindfulness-based exposure therapy can alleviate PTSD symptoms by redirecting attention from disturbing flashbacks to a focus on the present. Mindfulness based meditation practice has also been shown to increase attention and working memory in patients with mild traumatic brain injury (mTBI) or postconcussion syndrome and to strengthen the brain's ability to control emotions and reduce mood swings and anxiety.

CONCLUSION

Research demonstrating the brain's remarkable ability to overcome adversity offers promise for neurological recovery from child maltreatment with the appropriate interventions. Positive attachment relationships are essential in helping to heal trauma and buffer its negative effects. Building the capacity of birth, foster, kin, and adoptive parents to provide responsive caregiving to the children in their care (the National Scientific Council on the Developing Child, 2016)—as well as ensuring access to early intervention and trauma-informed practices—can help promote healthier brain development and improve outcomes for children, youth, and families involved in the child welfare system.

Chapter 36 | Help Your Child Be Successful at School after a TBI

WHAT IS A TRAUMATIC BRAIN INJURY?

A Traumatic Brain Injury (TBI) disrupts the normal functioning of the brain. A bump, a blow, or a jolt to the head can cause a TBI. With the brain still developing, a child is at greater risk for long-term effects after a TBI. These injuries range from mild to severe. Mild TBI, referred to as "mTBI" or "concussion," is most common.

COORDINATION IS THE KEY

Children recovering from a TBI need ongoing monitoring with coordinated care and support for best outcomes. Parents and families are often the ones taking care of children as they grow and develop.

Communicate

- Talk with your child's healthcare provider regularly, and attend all follow-up appointments.
- Notify your child's school about the TBI, and share updates from their healthcare provider.
- Communicate with the school about the need to monitor your child, and inform you about changes in your child's behavior or schoolwork.

This chapter includes text excerpted from "Help Your Child Be Successful at School after a TBI," Centers for Disease Control and Prevention (CDC), February 21, 2018.

Monitor
- Observe your child's symptoms and school work. Report concerns to your child's healthcare provider and school staff.
- Keep records about your child's head injuries, recovery, and recommendations from your doctor about services for your child, such as speech therapy.
- Watch for signs of changes in your child's behavior or school performance, as these may not show up right after a TBI.
- Keep track of the number of brain injuries your child has experienced, and consider this when making decisions about participation in activities like contact sports.

Help Your Child Return to School
Most students who return to school after a TBI benefit from a short-term plan that includes individualized accommodations, such as:
- Physical rest
- Extra time on tests
- Reduced homework load
- More frequent breaks
- Individualized help at school

FIND SUPPORT FOR YOUR FAMILY
Understanding the effects of a TBI on your child, and finding the right services to meet their needs can be a gradual process. It also may be important to find care for yourself through support groups or other services available in your community.

Connect
Support groups provide encouragement and valuable help for parents and caregivers.
- Parent Training Information Centers (PACER Family-to-Family Health Information Centers: www.pacer.org/about/PACERfacts.asp)

- Brain Injury Association of America (BIAA): www. biausa.org
- United States Brain Injury Alliance (USBIA): www. usbia.org
- National Association of State Head Injury Administrators (NASHIA): www.nashia.org

Engage

Problem-solving therapy (PST) can help families and children cope with a TBI. In PST, families receive training in:

- Staying positive
- Step-by-step problem-solving
- Family communication skills
- Education about the effects of a TBI

Chapter 37 | **Caring for a Person with Traumatic Brain Injury**

Family caregivers play an important role in recovery. In fact, many people who work with traumatic brain injury (TBI) patients believe that having a family caregiver is one of the most important aids to recovery. You can offer support, encouragement, and guidance to your injured family member, and help ensure the treatment plan established by the medical professionals caring for the veteran is followed.

At times, you may feel overwhelmed, angry, or scared. You may also feel alone, or feel worn out by caregiving responsibilities. These reactions are normal and typically come and go. If you feel like there is just too much to deal with, seek help either by confiding in a friend, participating in a support group, or consulting a professional mental-health practitioner.

CAREGIVING TIPS
- It is often difficult for an individual with TBI to multitask, so give one instruction at a time. Try using lists and memory notebooks. A calendar is also a helpful tool to organize daily tasks.
- Be sensitive to the issue of fatigue. If your family member seems tired or overwhelmed, suggest they take a break.

This chapter includes text excerpted from "Family Caregivers Guide to TBI: VA Caregiver Support," U.S. Department of Veterans Affairs (VA), May 2011. Reviewed May 2020.

- Establish a routine in which your family member preplans activities for the day. Scheduling the most important activities for the morning is a good idea, because energy levels tend to decline over the course of the day. Remember that your loved one will have good days and bad days, both emotionally and physically. This is a normal part of recovery.
- Know what resources are available and reach out to friends, family, and professionals. The U.S. Department of Veterans Affairs (VA) can help you learn about available resources at (www.caregiver.va.gov).
- Attend visits to the medical provider with your family member and provide detailed information about the veteran's progress and challenges. Ask questions and take notes.
- Be supportive and patient, but also remember to take care of yourself. If you find yourself completely overwhelmed or you feel yourself "losing it," take a moment and call someone—a friend, a family member, or VA's Caregiver Support Line (855-260-3274) are all good places to start. Support groups may also be available in your community or at your local VA.
- Visit your doctor regularly, and get plenty of rest so you can stay strong. Remember, you are doing the best you can and you are making a difference in your loved one's life.

Chapter 38 | **Returning to Sports and Activities after a Concussion**

After a concussion, an athlete should only return to sports practices with the approval and under the supervision of their healthcare provider. When available, be sure to also work closely with your team's certified athletic trainer.

Below are six gradual steps that you, along with a healthcare provider, should follow to help safely return an athlete to play. Remember, this is a gradual process. These steps should not be completed in one day, but instead over days, weeks, or months.

SIX-STEP RETURN TO PLAY PROGRESSION

It is important for an athlete's parent(s) and coach(es) to watch for concussion symptoms after each day's return to play progression activity. An athlete should only move to the next step if they do not have any new symptoms at the current step. If an athlete's symptoms come back or if she or he gets new symptoms, this is a sign that the athlete is pushing too hard. The athlete should stop these activities and the athlete's medical provider should be contacted. After more rest and no concussion symptoms, the athlete can start at the previous step.

This chapter includes text excerpted from "Returning to Sports and Activities," Centers for Disease Control and Prevention (CDC), February 12, 2019.

Step 1: Back to Regular Activities

Athletes are back to their regular activities (such as school) and has the green-light from their healthcare provider to begin the return to play process. An athlete's return to regular activities involves a stepwise process. It starts with a few days of rest (two to three days) and is followed by light activity (such as short walks) and moderate activity (such as riding a stationary bike) that do not worsen symptoms.

Step 2: Light Aerobic Activity

Begin with light aerobic exercise only to increase an athlete's heart rate. This means about 5 to 10 minutes on an exercise bike, walking, or light jogging. No weight lifting at this point.

Step 3: Moderate Activity

Continue with activities to increase an athlete's heart rate with body or head movement. This includes moderate jogging, brief running, moderate-intensity stationary biking, moderate-intensity weight-lifting (less time and/or less weight from their typical routine).

Step 4: Heavy, Noncontact Activity

Add heavy noncontact physical activity such as sprinting/running, high-intensity stationary biking, regular weightlifting routine, non-contact sport-specific drills (in three planes of movement).

Step 5: Practice and Full Contact

Young athletes may return to practice and full contact (if appropriate for the sport) in controlled practice.

Step 6: Competition

Young athletes may return to competition.

Chapter 39 | Factors Influencing Outcomes of Recovery

FACTORS INFLUENCING OUTCOMES

Recovery from traumatic brain injury (TBI) is influenced by classes of factors such as individual patient characteristics, social-environmental factors (e.g., family support systems), and barriers to rehabilitation access. The chapter outlines some of these specific factors.

Individual Characteristics

Individual characteristics, such as age and preinjury functioning, can influence outcomes after TBI. These characteristics differentially influence outcomes based upon the severity of injury. For example, children who sustain a moderate-to-severe TBI before 7 years of age have substantially worse short- and long-term outcomes than children who suffer a similar injury at an older age. Behavioral changes and problems in adaptive functioning (i.e., coping skills) are the most persistent negative impacts of TBI in children. Older adults who sustain a TBI have lower survival rates and less favorable outcomes than those who sustain a TBI during young and middle adulthood.

Preinjury functioning also is related to various cognitive and behavioral outcomes. People with higher levels of preinjury

This chapter includes text excerpted from "Report to Congress—Traumatic Brain Injury In the United States: Epidemiology and Rehabilitation," Centers for Disease Control and Prevention (CDC), June 15, 2013. Reviewed May 2020.

cognitive functioning often preserve more functional capacity after TBI. This hypothesis suggests that a person might be able to use cognitive resources postinjury that were not needed or used before the injury. Finally, growing evidence of the role of genetic influences on outcome suggests that some alleles, or gene variants, might confer neuro-protection to some and vulnerability to others post-TBI.

Social-Environmental Factors

Social-environmental factors such as socioeconomic status, caregiver and family functioning, and social support influence the effectiveness of rehabilitation treatments. Returning to participation in preinjury social roles also is an important aspect of functioning for adults after a TBI. The ability to function in social roles is related to psychological and neurocognitive outcomes, but can also be influenced by other factors, such as caregiver and family support, independent of TBI severity. Social-environmental factors such as the ability to live independently, maintain employment, or be involved in meaningful interpersonal relationships, such as marriage, also can influence outcomes for people affected by TBI.

Family-level factors are critical social-environmental influences on outcomes for children following a TBI. Family-level factors can include caregiver distress or depression, and deteriorating family functioning. Aspects of the home environment such as parental responsiveness, negativity, and discipline practices, are linked to a child's behavioral recovery. Economic and social disadvantages have been associated with poor cognitive and academic outcomes following severe TBI. Well-functioning caregivers and available financial and social supports contribute to better recovery and outcomes. In fact, family-centered interventions have been shown to be beneficial. Research has shown improved behavior of pediatric TBI patients and improved family functioning from this type of intervention. Studies also have demonstrated that cognitive-behavioral, problem-solving therapy can improve several pediatric outcomes, including executive function skills, behavior, and caregiver distress.

Access to Care after Hospitalization

People with TBI who transition from acute injury care often are discharged home or admitted to one of various rehabilitation programs or facilities. Discharge disposition is influenced by both clinical and nonclinical factors. These factors frequently influence the type and quantity of rehabilitation care received, which can affect TBI outcomes. In some instances, adults with moderate-to-severe TBI are discharged home where the level and intensity of rehabilitation is not well defined. For people who do not immediately return home, the decision to discharge patients to inpatient rehabilitation (i.e., postacute rehabilitation) or outpatient rehabilitation programs (i.e., subacute rehabilitation) is complex because the decision is frequently influenced by age, comorbidities, concurrent injuries, financial resources, and injury severity. Outpatient rehabilitation programs are less intense, and are composed of fewer total hours of therapy, on average, compared with inpatient rehabilitation.

Type of insurance coverage also is a predictor of discharge disposition. For example, the Centers for Medicare & Medicaid Services (CMS) established specific criteria in regulation for inpatient rehabilitation admission in order to fulfill statutory coverage requirements that inpatient rehabilitation facility claims for reasonable and necessary services. A patient's condition must require active and ongoing therapy by at least three separate disciplines, and the patient must be capable of participating in at least 3 hours of therapy, 5 days per week, or 15 hours during a 7-day period (the Centers for Medicare & Medicaid Services, 2012). In addition, a patient must also be reasonably expected to actively participate in, and benefit significantly from the intensive rehabilitation therapy program. Further, face-to-face supervision by a rehabilitation physician is required at least 3 days per week, and an intensive and coordinated interdisciplinary team approach to the delivery of rehabilitative care is also required. Patients who do not meet these criteria are discharged home or to subacute rehabilitation. Also, research suggests that patients with Medicare are more likely to be discharged to inpatient or outpatient rehabilitation (versus home) compared with patients who pay out of pocket. Outcomes for people with TBI can be influenced by any of these external factors regardless of injury severity. Additional research is required to understand the predictors of discharge disposition for people with moderate-to-severe TBI and the subsequent bearing on outcomes.

Chapter 40 | **Support Services for People with Traumatic Brain Injuries**

A traumatic brain injury (TBI) can happen when an external force causes severe damage to the brain. Common causes of TBI include falls, automobile accidents, and sports injuries. There are many different names for TBI such as concussion, shaken baby syndrome, head injury, or anoxia (loss of oxygen) due to trauma. Data from the National Institute on Disability, Independent Living, and Rehabilitation Research (NIDILRR)-supported research finds 1.56 million TBIs sustained in one year.

Traumatic brain injury can affect many parts of a person's life. People living with TBI and their families often require a range of services and support. Individual needs are different and can change over time, so it is important that systems provide person-centered services and supports.

ABOUT THE TRAUMATIC BRAIN INJURY STATE PARTNERSHIP GRANT PROGRAM

The TBI State Partnership Grant Program provides funding to help states increase access to services and support for individuals with TBI throughout their lifetime. This grant program is one component of the federal TBI Program, along with protection and advocacy systems (P&As), which is expected to:

This chapter includes text excerpted from "Traumatic Brain Injury (TBI) State Partnership Grant Program," Administration for Community Living (ACL), April 11, 2019.

- Help states expand and improve state and local capability so individuals with TBI and their families have better access to comprehensive and coordinated services.
- Generate support from local and private sources for sustainability of funded projects after federal support terminates. This is done through state legislative, regulatory, or policy changes that promote the integration of TBI-related services into state service delivery systems.
- Encourage systems to change activities so that individual states can 1) evaluate their current structures and policies and 2) improve their systems as needed to better meet the needs of individuals with TBI and their families.

AUTHORIZING LEGISLATION

The current authorizing legislation is the Traumatic Brain Injury Program Reauthorization Act of 2018 (P.L 115-377; (42 U.S.C. 300d–52)). It raised the authorization levels for the TBI State Partnership Program and TBI P&A and officially designated the Administration for Community Living (ACL) as the administering agency for both programs. Also, the new provision for partners at the Centers for Disease Control and Prevention (CDC) will allow them to implement and analyze concussion prevalence and incidence data, filling a longstanding data gap that will bolster all TBI programs.

TRAUMATIC BRAIN INJURY PROGRAMS TRANSITION TO ADMINISTRATION FOR COMMUNITY LIVING

The TBI Reauthorization Act of 2014 allowed the Department of Health and Human Services (HHS) Secretary to review oversight of the federal TBI Program and reconsider which administration should lead it. With support from TBI stakeholders, the Secretary found that the federal TBI Programs' goals closely align with the ACL's mission to advance policy and implement programs that support the rights of older Americans and people with disabilities to live in their communities. As a result, the federal TBI Program moved from the Health Resources and Services Administration (HRSA) to ACL on October 1, 2015.

STATE GRANTEE INFORMATION
Grants to States

Federal TBI Program grants to states have undergone several changes since the TBI Act of 1996 mandated the program. The most recent state grants were awarded in 2014 and require that grant activities increase access to rehabilitation and other services. Specifically, the states must address four barriers to needed services by:

- Screening to identify individuals with TBI
- Building a trained TBI workforce by providing professional training
- Providing information about TBI to families and referrals to appropriate service providers
- Facilitating access to needed services through resource facilitation

State Partnership Grants (SPGs) cannot be used to support primary injury prevention initiatives, research initiatives, or the provision of direct services. Funds may be used, however, to educate the public about the causes, symptoms, and treatment of TBI.

Between 1997 and 2018, 48 states, two territories, and the District of Columbia (DOC) received at least one state agency grant.

Traumatic Brain Injury Coordinating Center

In January 2019, the ACL asked for submissions of thoughts and ideas from TBI stakeholders regarding the future contract for the TBI Technical Assistance and Resource Center (TBI TARC). The ACL received thirteen submissions with recommendations. Here are some of the common themes from these responses as well as the full text redacted for identifying information.

The TBI Coordinating Center helps demonstrate the federal TBI Program's success in providing long-term benefits to public health and provides grantees access to resources that will help them build partnerships, promote positive outcomes, increase access, and build capacity.

The TBI Coordinating Center:

- Provides grantees with individualized technical assistance to help plan and develop effective programs that improve access to health and other services for individuals with TBI and their families
- Shares promising practices and lessons learned on implementing project activities and creating and/or incorporating TBI services, funding, etc.
- Communicates TBI-related information and research findings
- Offers best practices and tools for grantees to conduct state needs and resource assessments
- Responds to questions about the federal TBI Program and facilitates participation in program-related events

Legislation

Recognizing the large number of individuals and families struggling to access appropriate and community-based services, Congress authorized the federal TBI Program in the TBI Act of 1996 (PL 104-166). The TBI Act of 1996 launched an effort to conduct expanded studies and to establish innovative programs for TBI. The Act gave the Health Resources and Services Administration (HRSA) authority to establish a grant program for states to assist it in addressing the needs of individuals with TBI and their families. The TBI Act also delegated responsibilities in research to the National Institutes of Health (NIH), and prevention and surveillance to the CDC.

The Traumatic Brain Injury Act of 2008 (P.L. 110-206) reauthorized the programs of the TBI Act of 1996. The 2000 Amendments (PL 106-310—Title XIII of the Children's Health Act) recognized the importance of P&A services for individuals with TBI and their families by authorizing TBI Technical Assistance and Resource

Center to make grants to federally mandated state protection and advocacy systems. As a result of the TBI Reauthorization Act of 2014, the TBI Program transitioned from HRSA to ACL on October 1, 2015. The fiscal year 2015 appropriation was $9.321 million.

Part 7 | **Clinical Trials and Research Studies on Traumatic Brain Injury**

Chapter 41 | **Understanding Clinical Trials**

Section 41.1 | **What Are Clinical Trials and Studies?**

This section includes text excerpted from "What Are Clinical Trials and Studies?" National Institute on Aging (NIA), National Institutes of Health (NIH), April 9, 2020.

Clinical research is medical research involving people. There are two types, observational studies and clinical trials.

Observational studies observe people in normal settings. Researchers gather information, group volunteers according to broad characteristics, and compare changes over time. For example, researchers may collect data through medical exams, tests, or questionnaires about a group of older adults over time to learn more about the effects of different lifestyles on cognitive health. These studies may help identify new possibilities for clinical trials.

Clinical trials are research studies performed in people that are aimed at evaluating a medical, surgical, or behavioral intervention. They are the primary way that researchers find out if a new treatment, like a new drug or diet or medical device (for example, a pacemaker) is safe and effective in people. Often a clinical trial is used to learn if a new treatment is more effective and/or has less harmful side effects than the standard treatment.

Other clinical trials test ways to find a disease early, sometimes before there are symptoms. Still, others test ways to prevent a health problem. A clinical trial may also look at how to make life better for people living with a life-threatening disease or a chronic health problem. Clinical trials sometimes study the role of caregivers or support groups.

Before the U.S. Food and Drug Administration (FDA) approves a clinical trial to begin, scientists perform laboratory tests and studies in animals to test a potential therapy's safety and efficacy. If these studies show favorable results, the FDA gives approval for the intervention to be tested in humans.

WHAT ARE THE FOUR PHASES OF CLINICAL TRIALS?

Clinical trials advance through four phases to test a treatment, find the appropriate dosage, and look for side effects. If, after the first three phases, researchers find a drug or other intervention to be

311

safe and effective, the FDA approves it for clinical use and continues to monitor its effects.

Clinical trials of drugs are usually described based on their phase. The FDA typically requires Phase I, II, and III trials to be conducted to determine if the drug can be approved for use.

- A Phase I trial tests an experimental treatment on a small group of often healthy people (20 to 80) to judge its safety and side effects and to find the correct drug dosage.
- A Phase II trial uses more people (100 to 300). While the emphasis in Phase I is on safety, the emphasis in Phase II is on effectiveness. This phase aims to obtain preliminary data on whether the drug works in people who have a certain disease or condition. These trials also continue to study safety, including short-term side effects. This phase can last several years.
- A Phase III trial gathers more information about safety and effectiveness, studying different populations and different dosages, using the drug in combination with other drugs. The number of subjects usually ranges from several hundred to about 3,000 people. If the FDA agrees that the trial results are positive, it will approve the experimental drug or device.
- A Phase IV trial for drugs or devices takes place after the FDA approves their use. A device or drug's effectiveness and safety are monitored in large, diverse populations. Sometimes, the side effects of a drug may not become clear until more people have taken it over a longer period of time.

WHY PARTICIPATE IN A CLINICAL TRIAL?

There are many reasons why people choose to join a clinical trial. Some join a trial because the treatments they have tried for their health problem did not work. Others participate because there is no treatment for their health problem. By being part of a clinical trial, participants may find out about new treatments before they are widely available. Some studies are designed for, or include, people who are healthy but want to help find ways to prevent a disease, such as one that may be common in their family.

Many people say participating in a clinical trial is a way to play a more active role in their own healthcare. Other people say they want to help researchers learn more about certain health problems. Whatever the motivation, when you choose to participate in a clinical trial, you become a partner in scientific discovery. And, your contribution can help future generations lead healthier lives. Major medical breakthroughs could not happen without the generosity of clinical trial participants—young and old.

Here is what happens in a trial:

- Study staff explain the trial in detail and gather more information about you.
- Once you have had all your questions answered and agree to participate, you sign an informed consent form.
- You are screened to make sure you qualify for the trial.
- If accepted into the trial, you schedule a first visit (called the "baseline" visit). The researchers conduct cognitive and/or physical tests during this visit.
- You are randomly assigned to a treatment or control group.
- You and your family members follow the trial procedures and report any issues or concerns to researchers.
- You may visit the research site at regularly scheduled times for new cognitive, physical, or other evaluations and discussions with staff. At these visits, the research team collects information about effects of the intervention and your safety and well-being.
- You continue to see your regular physician for usual healthcare throughout the study.

Where Can I Find a Clinical Trial?

There are many ways you can get help to find a clinical trial. You can talk to your doctor or other healthcare provider. Or, you can search ClinicalTrials.gov. You can sign up for a registry or matching service to connect you with trials in your area. Support groups and websites that focus on a particular condition sometimes have lists of clinical studies. Also, you may see ads for trials in your area in the newspaper or on TV.

What Is the Next Step after I Find a Clinical Trial?

Once you find a study that you might want to join, contact the clinical trial or study coordinator. You can usually find this contact information in the description of the study. The first step is a screening appointment to see if you qualify to participate. This appointment also gives you a chance to ask your questions about the study.

Let your doctor know that you are thinking about joining a clinical trial. She or he may want to talk to the research team about your health to make sure the study is safe for you and to coordinate your care while you are in the study.

How Do Researchers Decide Who Will Participate?

After you consent, you will be screened by clinical staff to see if you meet the criteria to participate in the trial or if anything would exclude you. The screening may involve cognitive and physical tests.

Inclusion criteria for a trial might include age, stage of disease, sex, genetic profile, family history, and whether or not you have a study partner who can accompany you to future visits. Exclusion criteria might include factors such as specific health conditions or medications that could interfere with the treatment being tested.

Many volunteers must be screened to find enough people for a study. Generally, you can participate in only one trial or study at a time. Different trials have different criteria, so being excluded from one trial does not necessarily mean exclusion from another.

WHY ARE OLDER AND DIVERSE PARTICIPANTS IMPORTANT IN CLINICAL TRIALS?

It is important for clinical trials to have participants of different ages, sexes, races, and ethnicities. When research involves a group of people who are similar, the findings may not apply to or benefit everyone. When clinical trials include diverse participants, the study results may have a much wider applicability.

Researchers need the participation of older people in their clinical trials so that scientists can learn more about how the new drugs, therapies, medical devices, surgical procedures, or tests will work for older people. Many older people have special health needs that are different from those of younger people. For example, as people age, their bodies may react differently to drugs. Older adults may need different dosages (or amounts) of a drug to have the right result. Also, some drugs may have different side effects in older people than younger people. Having seniors enrolled in drug trials helps researchers get the information they need to develop the right treatment for older people.

Researchers know that it may be hard for some older people to join a clinical trial. For example, if you have many health problems, can you participate in a trial that is looking at only one condition? If you are frail or have a disability, will you be strong enough to participate? If you no longer drive, how can you get to the study site? Talk to the clinical trial coordinator about your concerns. The research team may have already thought about some of the obstacles for older people and have a plan to make it easier for you to take part in the trial.

QUESTIONS TO ASK BEFORE PARTICIPATING IN A CLINICAL TRIAL

The following are some questions to ask the research team when thinking about a clinical trial. Write down any questions you might have and bring your list with you when you first meet with the research team.

About the Trial
- What is this study trying to find out?
- What treatment or tests will I have? Will they hurt? Will you give me the test or lab results?
- What are the chances I will get the experimental treatment or the placebo?

- What are the possible risks, side effects, and benefits of the study treatment compared with my current treatment?
- How will I know if the treatment is working?
- How long will the clinical trial last?
- Where will the study take place? Will I have to stay in the hospital?
- Will you provide a way for me to get to the study site if I need it, such as a rideshare service?
- Can I do any part of the trial with my regular doctor? Is there a closer clinical trial to me?
- How will the study affect my everyday life?
- What steps ensure my privacy?

Medical Care
- How will you protect my health while I am in the study?
- What happens if my health problem gets worse during the study?
- Can I take my regular medicines while in the trial?
- Who will be in charge of my care while I am in the study? Will I be able to see my own doctor?
- How will you keep my doctor informed about my participation in the trial?
- If I withdraw, will this affect my normal care?

Costs and Reimbursement
- Will being in the study cost me anything? If so, will I be reimbursed for expenses such as travel, parking, or lodging?
- Will my insurance pay for costs not covered by the research trial, or will I need to pay out of pocket? If I do not have insurance, am I still eligible to participate?
- Will I need a study partner? If so, how long will she or he need to participate? Will my study partner be compensated for her or his time?

After the Trial Ends
- Will you follow-up on my health after the end of the study?
- Will you tell me the results of the study?
- Whom do I call if I have more questions?

Section 41.2 | Participating in Clinical Studies

This section contains text excerpted from the following sources: Text in this section begins with excerpts from "Learn about Clinical Studies," ClinicalTrials.gov, National Institutes of Health (NIH), March 2019; Text under the heading "Finding a Clinical Trial" is excerpted from "Finding a Clinical Trial," National Institutes of Health (NIH), November 6, 2018.

A clinical study is conducted according to a research plan known as the "protocol." The protocol is designed to answer specific research questions and safeguard the health of participants. It contains the following information:
- The reason for conducting the study
- Who may participate in the study (the eligibility criteria)
- The number of participants needed
- The schedule of tests, procedures, or drugs and their dosages
- The length of the study
- What information will be gathered about the participants

WHO CAN PARTICIPATE IN A CLINICAL STUDY?
Clinical studies have standards outlining who can participate. These standards are called "eligibility criteria" and are listed in the protocol. Some research studies seek participants who have the illnesses or conditions that will be studied; other studies are looking for healthy participants; and some studies are limited to a predetermined group of people who are asked by researchers to enroll.

317

Eligibility. The factors that allow someone to participate in a clinical study are called "inclusion criteria," and the factors that disqualify someone from participating are called "exclusion criteria." They are based on characteristics such as age, gender, the type and stage of a disease, previous treatment history, and other medical conditions.

HOW ARE PARTICIPANTS PROTECTED?

Informed consent is a process used by researchers to provide potential and enrolled participants with information about a clinical study. This information helps people decide whether they want to enroll or continue to participate in the study. The informed consent process is intended to protect participants and should provide enough information for a person to understand the risks of, potential benefits of, and alternatives to the study. In addition to the informed consent document, the process may involve recruitment materials, verbal instructions, question-and-answer sessions, and activities to measure participant understanding. In general, a person must sign an informed consent document before joining a study to show that she or he was given information on the risks, potential benefits and alternatives, and that she or he understands it. Signing the document and providing consent is not a contract. Participants may withdraw from a study at any time, even if the study is not over.

Institutional review boards. Each federally supported or conducted clinical study and each study of a drug, biological product, or medical device regulated by the U.S. Food and Drug Administration (FDA) must be reviewed, approved, and monitored by an institutional review board (IRB). An IRB is made up of doctors, researchers, and members of the community. Its role is to make sure that the study is ethical and that the rights and welfare of participants are protected. This includes making sure that research risks are minimized and are reasonable in relation to any potential benefits, among other responsibilities. The IRB also reviews the informed consent document.

In addition to being monitored by an IRB, some clinical studies are also monitored by data monitoring committees (also called "data safety" and "monitoring boards").

Various federal agencies, including the Office of Human Subjects Research Protection and FDA, have the authority to determine whether sponsors of certain clinical studies are adequately protecting research participants.

RELATIONSHIP TO USUAL HEALTHCARE

Typically, participants continue to see their usual healthcare providers while enrolled in a clinical study. While most clinical studies provide participants with medical products or interventions related to the illness or condition being studied, they do not provide extended or complete healthcare. By having her or his usual healthcare provider work with the research team, a participant can make sure that the study protocol will not conflict with other medications or treatments that she or he receives.

CONSIDERATIONS FOR PARTICIPATION

Participating in a clinical study contributes to medical knowledge. The results of these studies can make a difference in the care of future patients by providing information about the benefits and risks of therapeutic, preventative, or diagnostic products or interventions.

Clinical trials provide the basis for the development and marketing of new drugs, biological products, and medical devices. Sometimes, the safety and the effectiveness of the experimental approach or use may not be fully known at the time of the trial. Some trials may provide participants with the prospect of receiving direct medical benefits, while others do not. Most trials involve some risk of harm or injury to the participant, although it may not be greater than the risks related to routine medical care or disease progression. (For trials approved by IRBs, the IRB has decided that the risks of participation have been minimized and are reasonable in relation to anticipated benefits.) Many trials require participants to undergo additional procedures, tests, and assessments based on the study protocol. These requirements will be described in the informed consent document. A potential participant should also discuss these issues with members of the research team and with her or his usual healthcare provider.

QUESTIONS TO ASK

Anyone interested in participating in a clinical study should know as much as possible about the study and feel comfortable asking the research team questions about the study, the related procedures, and any expenses. The following questions may be helpful during such a discussion. Answers to some of these questions are provided in the informed consent document. Many of the questions are specific to clinical trials, but some also apply to observational studies.

- What is being studied?
- Why do researchers believe the intervention being tested might be effective? Why might it not be effective? Has it been tested before?
- What are the possible interventions that I might receive during the trial?
- How will it be determined which interventions I receive (for example, by chance)?
- Who will know which intervention I receive during the trial? Will I know? Will members of the research team know?
- How do the possible risks, side effects, and benefits of this trial compare with those of my current treatment?
- What will I have to do?
- What tests and procedures are involved?
- How often will I have to visit the hospital or clinic?
- Will hospitalization be required?
- How long will the study last?
- Who will pay for my participation?
- Will I be reimbursed for other expenses?
- What type of long-term follow-up care is part of this trial?
- If I benefit from the intervention, will I be allowed to continue receiving it after the trial ends?
- Will results of the study be provided to me?
- Who will oversee my medical care while I am participating in the trial?
- What are my options if I am injured during the study?

FINDING A CLINICAL TRIAL
Around the Nation and Worldwide

The National Institutes of Health (NIH) conducts clinical research trials for many diseases and conditions, including cancer, Alzheimer disease (AD), allergy and infectious diseases, and neurological disorders. To search for other diseases and conditions, you can visit ClinicalTrials.gov.

CLINICALTRIALS.GOV

This is a searchable registry and results database of federally and privately supported clinical trials conducted in the United States and around the world. ClinicalTrials.gov gives you information about a trial's purpose, who may participate, locations, and phone numbers for more details. This information should be used in conjunction with advice from healthcare professionals.

Listing a study does not mean it has been evaluated by the United States federal government.

Before participating in a study, talk to your healthcare provider and learn about the risks and potential benefits.

At the National Institutes of Health Clinical Center in Bethesda, Maryland
NATIONAL INSTITUTES OF HEALTH CLINICAL RESEARCH STUDIES

The NIH maintains an online database of clinical research studies taking place at its clinical center, which is located on the NIH campus in Bethesda, Maryland. Studies are conducted by most of the institutes and centers across the NIH. The clinical center hosts a wide range of studies from rare diseases to chronic health conditions, as well as studies for healthy volunteers. Visitors can search by diagnosis, signs, symptoms, or other key words.

Join a National Registry of Research Volunteers

This is an NIH-funded initiative to connect:
1. People who are trying to find research studies
2. Researchers seeking people to participate in their studies.

It is a free, secure registry to make it easier for the public to volunteer and to become involved in clinical research studies that contribute to improved health in the future.

Chapter 42 | **Research Studies on Traumatic Brain Injury**

Chapter Contents

Section 42.1 | Supporting Research Studies for Better Treatment Options

This section includes text excerpted from "Traumatic Brain Injury: Hope through Research," National Institute of Neurological Disorders and Stroke (NINDS), April 24, 2020.

If you or someone you know has been diagnosed with a traumatic brain injury (TBI), enrolling in a clinical trial or brain bank are the best ways to support research toward new and better treatment options.

Clinical trials are research studies that involve people. Studies involving individuals with TBI and healthy individuals offer researchers the opportunity to greatly increase the National Institute of Neurological Disorders and Stroke's (NINDS) knowledge of TBI and find better ways to safely detect, treat, and ultimately prevent TBI. By participating in a clinical study, healthy individuals and those with TBI can greatly benefit the lives of those living with this disorder. Talk with your doctor about clinical studies and help to make the difference in the quality of life (QOL) for all people with TBI. Trials take place at medical centers across the United States and elsewhere.

People with a TBI also can support TBI research by designating the donation of brain tissue before they die. The study of human brain tissue is essential to increasing the understanding of how the nervous system functions.

The National Institutes of Health (NIH) NeuroBioBank is an effort by the NIH to coordinate the network of brain banks it supports in the United States to facilitate advances in research through the collection and distribution of postmortem brain tissue. Stakeholder groups include brain and tissue repositories, researchers, NIH program staff, information technology experts, disease advocacy groups, and most importantly individuals seeking information about opportunities to donate. It ensures protection of the privacy and wishes of donors. Creating a network of these centers makes it more likely that precious tissue can be made available to the greatest number of scientists.

Section 42.2 | Tiny Bleeds Associated with Disability after Brain Injury

This section includes text excerpted from "Tiny Bleeds Associated with Disability after Brain Injury," National Institutes of Health (NIH), October 29, 2019.

More than two million people nationwide suffer a traumatic brain injury (TBI) every year. Causes include motor vehicle accidents, falls, and violence. Although most people with a TBI will recover, over three million currently live with some level of disability caused by their injury.

The initial severity of a brain injury does not always predict who will experience disability. Many people with a TBI classified as mild still have life-long effects from their injury.

Researchers have wondered if a type of tiny abnormality seen on MRI in some people with TBI may be associated with long-term disability. Some scientists proposed that these tiny spots or lines, called "traumatic microbleeds" (TMBs), are caused by the tearing of nerve cells in the brain. Others suggested that they represent damage to blood vessels. The relationship between TMBs and long-term disability has been unclear.

To examine this relationship more closely, a research team led by Dr. Lawrence Latour from NIH's National Institute of Neurological Disorders and Stroke (NINDS) used MRI to examine the brains of 439 people who were admitted to trauma centers with a TBI. Participants underwent MRI imaging within 48 hours of their initial injury. About half also returned for follow-up scans, up to 3 months afterwards.

The researchers compared the risk of disability between people with and without TMBs. One participant died of an unrelated cause seven months after his initial magnetic resonance imaging (MRI), and his family donated his brain to the study. The scientists used the brain to compare actual tissue changes to TMB spots and lines seen on his MRI images.

The study was funded in part by NINDS and the NIH Clinical Center. Results were published on October 14, 2019, in *Brain*.

About 31 percent of all participants had TMBs on their MRI scans. These abnormalities were not confined to people with severe brain injuries: 27 percent of people with mild TBI and 47 percent of people with moderate TBI had evidence of TMBs.

People with TMBs immediately after their injury were twice as likely to report disability 30 and 90 days afterwards than people with no TMBs. Microbleeds were associated with disability independent of other known risk factors, including severity of the overall brain injury and damage seen on computed tomography (CT) scans.

Imaging and dissection of the donated brain found evidence of damage to the blood vessels at the sites of TMBs. The researchers did not see the nerve cell damage. Because only one brain was available for tissue studies, the researchers could not rule out nerve cell damage playing a role in some TMBs.

The findings suggest that people with TMBs may be candidates for treatment with drugs that target damaged blood vessels.

"Traumatic microbleeds may represent injury to blood vessels that occur following even minor head injury," Latour says. "While we know that damage to brain cells can be devastating, the exact impact of this vascular injury following head trauma is uncertain and requires further study."

Section 42.3 | Many with Mild Traumatic Brain Injury Do Not Receive Follow-Up Care

This section includes text excerpted from "Many with Mild Traumatic Brain Injury Don't Receive Follow-Up Care," National Institutes of Health (NIH), June 12, 2018.

Millions of Americans go to the hospital each year for treatment of mild traumatic brain injury (TBI), also known as "concussion." Though rarely fatal, concussions can have long-term effects that decrease quality of life (QOL). These include headaches, trouble with memory and reasoning, difficulty sleeping, and depression. A recent study found that almost a quarter of people with mild TBI still have related physical or mental problems a year later.

Other studies have suggested that many patients with mild TBI do not receive follow-up care that could help them manage these problems. A team led by Dr. Seth A. Seabury at the University of southern California and Dr. Geoffrey Manley of the University of California, San Francisco, set out to better understand how such follow-up care is delivered nationwide. Using data from a large study of TBI patients called "TRACK-TBI," they followed 831 people who were treated for mild TBI at 11 major trauma centers across the country. All the participants had symptoms that triggered a computed tomography (CT) scan of their brain as part of initial treatment. Traffic incidents and falls accounted for most of the cases.

The participants were asked about their follow-up care using two surveys, collected two weeks and three months after their injury. They reported whether they had received educational materials about their TBI when leaving the hospital, if the hospital had called to check up on them, and if they had seen a doctor or other health-care practitioner since going home. The research was supported in part by NIH's National Institute of Neurological Disorders and Stroke (NINDS). Results were published in *JAMA Network Open* on May 25, 2018.

Overall, about 42 percent of the participants said they had received educational materials when leaving the hospital. Only 27 percent received a follow-up call from the hospital. Within three months of their injury, 44 percent had seen a healthcare professional. These percentages varied widely between hospitals. Centers with dedicated TBI clinics provided the highest rates of follow-up care.

People with more serious injuries were somewhat more likely to receive follow-up care. In 236 participants who had tissue damage on their initial CT scan, 61 percent had seen a medical practitioner by three months after their injury. However, 39 percent had not. Of the 279 participants who reported that they still had three or more moderate or severe symptoms from their concussion three months later, only about half had seen a doctor about those symptoms. Whether or not people had health insurance did not affect the rates of follow-up care.

"Even in the best trauma centers in the country, patients with concussion are not getting the follow-up care they desperately need," Manley says.

"This is a public health crisis that is being overlooked," he adds. "For too many patients, concussion is being treated as a minor injury."

Section 42.4 | Every Cell Has a Story to Tell in Brain Injury

This section includes text excerpted from "Every Cell Has a Story to Tell in Brain Injury," National Institutes of Health (NIH), October 3, 2018.

Traumatic head injury can have widespread effects in the brain, but now scientists can look in real time at how head injury affects thousands of individual cells and genes simultaneously in mice. This approach could lead to precise treatments for traumatic brain injury (TBI). The study, reported in *Nature Communications*, was supported by the National Institute of Neurological Disorders and Stroke (NINDS), part of the National Institutes of Health (NIH).

"Instead of clustering responses according to categories of cells in TBI, we can now see how individual cells in those groups react to head injury," said Patrick Bellgowan, Ph.D., program director at NINDS.

University of California, Los Angeles professors Fernando Gómez-Pinilla, Ph.D., and Xia Yang, Ph.D., along with their colleagues, used a novel method known as "Drop-seq" to closely look at individual brain cells in the hippocampus, a region involved in learning and memory, after TBI or in uninjured control animals. Drop-seq allows thousands of cells and genes to be analyzed simultaneously. Its creation was in part funded by the NIH's Brain Research through Advancing Innovative Neurotechnologies (BRAIN) Initiative.

"These tools provide us with unprecedented precision to pinpoint exactly which cells and genes to target with new therapies," said Dr. Yang. "Another important aspect to this study was the highly collaborative and multidisciplinary nature of the work. Lots of people, from many different scientific areas, made this study possible."

In one set of experiments the team looked at TBI's effects on gene expression activity in individual cells. They found that certain genes were upregulated or downregulated across many different cell types, suggesting these genes may play important roles in TBI. Some of these genes are also known to be involved in diseases, such as Alzheimer disease (AD), which may help explain how TBI can be a risk factor for other disorders. For example, Drs. Yang and Gomez-Pinilla's groups observed altered activity in genes that are involved in regulating the amyloid protein, which builds up in Alzheimer.

In particular, the genomic analysis revealed that the activity of the *Ttr* gene, which is involved in both thyroid hormone transport and scavenging of amyloid protein in the brain, was increased in many cells following TBI, suggesting that the thyroid hormone pathway may be a potential target for therapy. Drs. Gomez-Pinilla and Yang's teams treated animals with the thyroid hormone thyroxine (T4) 1 and 6 hours after brain injury and saw that they performed much better on learning and memory tasks compared to animals that received a placebo.

The team identified 15 clusters of cells based on gene activity, including two clusters, named Unknown1 and Unknown2, the cells of which had not been described previously in the hippocampus. Further analysis of these clusters revealed that the cells in the Unknown1 group were involved in cell growth and migration and the cells in Unknown2 were involved in cell differentiation during development. The findings in this study also reveal that although two cells may have similar structure and shape, their functions, as suggested by the analysis of gene activity, may differ.

"We now know the secret life of single cells, including how they coordinate with other cells and how vulnerable they are to injury," said Dr. Gomez-Pinilla. "In addition, seeing which types of genes, including genes involved in metabolism, were involved across many cell types helps identify processes that may be critical in TBI."

Part 8 | Additional Help and Information

Chapter 43 | Glossary of Terms Related to TBI

addiction: A chronic, relapsing disease characterized by compulsive drug seeking and use, despite serious adverse consequences, and by long-lasting changes in the brain.

antidepressant: Medication used to treat depression, and other mood and anxiety disorders.

axon: The long, fiber-like part of a neuron by which the cell sends information to receiving neurons.

blood clot: A mass of blood that forms when blood platelets, proteins, and cells stick together. When a blood clot is attached to the wall of a blood vessel, it is called a "thrombus."

brain death: A lack of measurable brain function activity and blood flow after an extended period of time.

chronic: Persisting for a long time or constantly recurring.

chronic traumatic encephalopathy (CTE): Brain damage caused by cumulative and repetitive head trauma.

clinical trial: A scientific study using human volunteers (also called "participants") to look at new ways to prevent, detect, or treat disease. Treatments might be new drugs or new combinations of drugs, new surgical procedures or devices, or new ways to use existing treatments.

cognition: Conscious mental activities (such as thinking, communicating, understanding, solving problems, processing information, and remembering) that are associated with gaining knowledge and understanding.

cognitive behavioral therapy (CBT): CBT helps people focus on how to solve their current problems. The therapist helps the patient learn how to

This glossary contains terms excerpted from documents produced by several sources deemed reliable.

identify distorted or unhelpful thinking patterns, recognize and change inaccurate beliefs, relate to others in more positive ways, and change behaviors accordingly.

cognitive rehabilitation therapy (CRT): A strategy aimed at helping individuals with severe traumatic brain injury (TBI) regain their normal brain function through an individualized training program.

coma: A state of profound unconsciousness caused by disease, injury, or poison.

computed tomography (CT): A scan that creates a series of cross-sectional x-rays of the head and brain; also called "computerized axial tomography" or "CAT scan."

concussion: Injury to the brain caused by a hard blow or violent shaking of the brain within the skull, which produces a sudden and temporary impairment of brain function such as amnesia, short loss of consciousness, or disturbance of vision and equilibrium.

contrecoup: A contusion caused by the shaking of the brain back and forth within the confines of the skull.

contusion: A distinct area of swollen or bruised brain tissue mixed with blood released from broken blood vessels.

coup injury: A head injury that occurs under the site of impact with an object.

deep vein thrombosis (DVT): Formation of a blood clot deep within a vein.

dementia: Loss of brain function that occurs with certain diseases. It affects memory, thinking, language, judgment, and behavior.

dendrite: The point of contact for receiving impulses on a neuron, branching off from the cell body.

dopamine: A brain chemical, classified as a neurotransmitter, found in regions that regulate movement, emotion, motivation, and pleasure.

dura: A tough, fibrous membrane lining the brain; the outermost of the three membranes is collectively called the "meninges."

fatigue: Loss of energy or strength.

genes: A gene is a part of deoxyribonucleic acid (DNA) (the genetic instructions in all living things). People inherit one copy of each gene from their mother and one copy from their father.

Glasgow Coma Scale (GCS): A clinical tool used to assess the degree of consciousness and neurological functioning, and therefore, severity of brain injury: by testing motor responsiveness, verbal acuity, and eye opening.

Glossary of Terms Related to TBI

hematoma: Heavy bleeding into or around the brain caused by damage to a major blood vessel in the head.

hippocampus: A portion of the brain involved in creating and filing new memories.

hypothalamus: A structure in the brain under the thalamus that monitors activities, such as body temperature and food intake.

inpatient: A person who has been admitted at least overnight to a hospital or other health facility (which is, therefore, responsible for her or his room and board) for the purpose of receiving diagnostic treatment or other health services.

intracranial pressure: Buildup of pressure in the brain as a result of injury.

magnetic resonance imaging (MRI): A noninvasive diagnostic technique that uses magnetic fields to detect subtle changes in brain tissue.

medicaid: Federal and state-funded program of medical assistance to low-income individuals of all ages.

meditation: A group of techniques, most of which started in Eastern religious or spiritual traditions. In meditation, individuals learn to focus their attention and suspend the stream of thoughts that normally occupy the mind. This practice is believed to result in a state of greater physical relaxation, mental calmness, and psychological balance. Practicing meditation can change how a person relates to the flow of emotions and thoughts in the mind.

nervous system: The nervous system controls everything that a person does such as breathing, moving, and, thinking. This system is made up of the brain, spinal cord, and all the nerves in the body.

neuron: A nerve cell that is the basic, working unit of the brain and nervous system, which processes and transmits information.

neurotransmitters: Chemicals that transmit nerve signals from one neuron to another.

penetrating head injury (or open head injury): A brain injury in which an object pierces the skull and enters the brain tissue.

posttraumatic epilepsy: Recurrent seizures occurring more than one week after a traumatic brain injury (TBI).

posttraumatic stress disorder (PTSD): An anxiety disorder that develops in reaction to physical injury or severe mental or emotional distress such as military combat, violent assault, natural disaster, or other life-threatening events.

psychologist: A clinical psychologist is a professional who treats mental illness, emotional disturbance, and behavior problems. They use talk therapy as treatment, and cannot prescribe medication. A clinical psychologist will have a master's degree (M.A.) or doctorate (Ph.D.) in psychology, and possibly more training in a specific type of therapy.

seizures: Abnormal activity of nerve cells in the brain causing strange sensations, emotions, and behavior, or sometimes convulsions, muscle spasms, and loss of consciousness.

shaken baby syndrome: A severe form of head injury that occurs when an infant or small child is shaken forcibly enough to cause the brain to bounce against the skull; the degree of brain damage depends on the extent and duration of the shaking. Minor symptoms include irritability, lethargy, tremors, or vomiting; major symptoms include seizures, coma, stupor, or death.

skull fractures: Breaks or cracks in one or more of the bones that form the skull, which can damage the underlying areas of the skull including the brain, membranes, and blood vessels.

stimulants: A class of drugs that enhances the activity of monamines (such as dopamine) in the brain, increasing arousal, heart rate, blood pressure, and respiration, and decreasing appetite; includes some medications used to treat attention deficit hyperactivity disorder (ADHD) (e.g., methylphenidate and amphetamines), as well as cocaine and methamphetamine.

subdural hematoma: Bleeding confined to the area between the dura and the arachnoid membranes.

synapse: The tiny gap between neurons, where nerve impulses are sent from one neuron to another.

thyroid hormone: A hormone that affects heart rate, blood pressure, body temperature, and weight. Thyroid hormone is made by the thyroid gland and can also be made in the laboratory.

tolerance: A condition in which higher doses of a drug are required to produce the same effect achieved during initial use; often associated with physical dependence.

vegetative state: A condition in which patients are unconscious and unaware of their surroundings, but continue to have a sleep/wake cycle and can have periods of alertness.

Chapter 44 | **Directory of TBI Organizations and Resources**

GOVERNMENT ORGANIZATIONS

Administration for Community Living (ACL)
330 C St., S.W.
Washington, DC 20201
Toll-Free: 800-677-1116
Phone: 202-401-4634
Website: www.acl.gov

Agency for Healthcare Research and Quality (AHRQ)
Office of Communications
5600 Fishers Ln.
Seventh Fl.
Rockville, MD 20847
Phone: 301-427-1104
Website: www.ahrq.gov

Brain Resources and Information Network (BRAIN)
National Institute of Neurological
Disorders and Stroke (NINDS)
P.O. Box 5801
Bethesda, MD 20824
Toll-Free: 800-352-9424
Phone: 301-496-5751
Fax: 301-402-2186
Website: www.ninds.nih.gov
E-mail: braininfo@ninds.nih.gov

Resources in this chapter were compiled from several sources deemed reliable; all contact information was verified and updated in May 2020.

Centers for Disease Control and Prevention (CDC)
1600 Clifton Rd.
Atlanta, GA 30329-4027
Toll-Free: 800-CDC-INFO
(800-232-4636)
Phone: 404-639-3311
Toll-Free TTY: 888-232-6348
Website: www.cdc.gov
E-mail: cdcinfo@cdc.gov

Child Welfare Information Gateway
Children's Bureau/Administration
on Children, Youth and Families
(ACYF)
330 C. S.W.
Washington, DC 20201
Toll-Free: 800-394-3366
Website: www.childwelfare.gov
E-mail: info@childwelfare.gov

Eunice Kennedy Shriver National Institute of Child Health and Human Development (NICHD)
NICHD Information Resource
Center (IRC)
P.O. Box 3006
Rockville, MD 20847
Toll-Free: 800-370-2943
Phone: 301-496-5133
Toll-Free Fax: 866-760-5947
Website: www.nichd.nih.gov
E-mail: NICHDInformation
ResourceCenter@mail.nih.gov

MedlinePlus
U.S. National Library of Medicine
(NLM)
8600 Rockville Pike
Bethesda, MD 20894
Toll-Free: 888-FIND-NLM
(888-346-3656)
Phone: 301-594-5983
Website: www.medlineplus.gov

National Highway Traffic Safety Administration (NHTSA)
1200 New Jersey Ave. S.E.
W. Bldg.
Washington, DC 20590
Toll-Free: 888-327-4236
Phone: 202-366-9550
Toll-Free TTY: 800-424-9153
Website: www.nhtsa.gov
E-mail: nhtsa.webmaster@dot.gov

National Institute of Neurological Disorders and Stroke (NINDS)
NIH Neurological Institute
P.O. Box 5801
Bethesda, MD 20824
Toll-Free: 800-352-9424
Website: www.ninds.nih.gov

National Institute on Aging (NIA)
31 Center Dr., MSC 2292
Bldg. 31, Rm. 5C27
Bethesda, MD 20892
Toll-Free: 800-222-2225
Toll-Free TTY: 800-222-4225
Website: www.nia.nih.gov
E-mail: niaic@nia.nih.gov

National Institute on Drug Abuse (NIDA)

Office of Science Policy and
Communications (OSPC)
6001 Executive Blvd.
Rm. 5213, MSC 9561
Bethesda, MD 20892
Phone: 301-443-1124
Website: www.drugabuse.gov

National Institutes of Health (NIH)

9000 Rockville Pike
Bethesda, MD 20892
Phone: 301-496-4000
Website: www.nih.gov

U.S. Department of Veterans Affairs (VA)

Toll-Free: 844-698-2311
Website: www.va.gov

U.S. Food and Drug Administration (FDA)

10903 New Hampshire Ave.
Silver Spring, MD 20993-0002
Toll-Free: 888-INFO-FDA
(888-463-6332)
Website: www.fda.gov

USA.gov

Toll-Free: 844-USA-GOV1
(844-872-4681)
Website: www.usa.gov

PRIVATE ORGANIZATIONS

Alzheimer's Foundation of America (AFA)

322 Eighth Ave.
16th Fl.
New York, NY 10001
Toll-Free: 866-232-8484
Fax: 646-638-1546
Website: www.alzfdn.org
E-mail: info@alzfdn.org

American Brain Tumor Association (ABTA)

8550 W. Bryn Mawr Ave., Ste. 550
Chicago, IL 60631
Toll-Free: 800-886-2282
Phone: 773-577-8750
Fax: 773-577-8738
Website: www.abta.org
E-mail: info@abta.org

American Parkinson Disease Association (APDA)

135 Parkinson Ave.
Staten Island, NY 10305
Toll-Free: 800-223-2732
Phone: 718-981-8001
Fax: 718-981-4399
Website: www.apdaparkinson.org/
contact
E-mail: apda@apdaparkinson.org

Brain & Behavior Research Foundation

747 Third Ave.
33rd Fl.
New York, NY 10017
Toll-Free: 800-829-8289
Phone: 646-681-4888
Website: www.bbrfoundation.org
E-mail: info@bbrfoundation.org

Brain Aneurysm Foundation (BAF)

269 Hanover St.
Bldg. 3
Hanover, MA 02339
Toll-Free: 888-272-4602
Phone: 781-826-5556
Fax: 781-826-5566
Website: bafound.org
E-mail: office@bafound.org

Brain Attack Coalition (BAC)

31 Center Dr., MSC 2540
Bldg. 31 Rm. 8A-07
Bethesda, MD 20892
Phone: 301-496-5751
Website: www.brainattackcoalition.org

Brain Injury Association of America (BIAA)

1608 Spring Hill Rd.
Ste. 110
Vienna, VA 22182
Toll-Free: 800-444-6443
Phone: 703-761-0750
Fax: 703-761-0755
Website: www.biausa.org
E-mail: info@biausa.org

The Brain Injury Recovery Network

840 Central Ave.
Carlisle, OH 45005
Toll-Free: 877-810-2100
Website: www.tbirecovery.org
E-mail: help@tbirecovery.org

Brain Injury Resource Center

P.O. Box 84151
Seattle, WA 98124-5451
Phone: 206-621-8558
Website: www.headinjury.com
E-mail: brain@headinjury.com

Brain Trauma Foundation (BTF)

228 Hamilton Ave.
Third Fl.
Palo Alto, CA 94301
Website: www.braintrauma.org

Child Neurology Foundation (CNF)

201 Chicago Ave. Ste. 200
Minneapolis, MN 55415
Phone: 612-928-6325
Website: www.childneurologyfoundation.org
E-mail: info@childneurologyfoundation.org

Epilepsy Foundation

8301 Professional Pl., W.
Landover, MD 20785-2356
Toll-Free: 800-EFA-1000
(800-332-1000)
Phone: 301-459-3700
Fax: 301-577-2684
Website: www.epilepsy.com
E-mail: ContactUs@efa.org

International Foundation for Research and Education on Depression (iFred)

P.O. Box 17598
Baltimore, MD 21297
Fax: 443-782-0739
Website: www.ifred.org
E-mail: info@ifred.org

International Society for Traumatic Stress Studies (ISTSS)

One Parkview Plaza.
Ste. 800
Oakbrook Terrace, IL 60181
Phone: 847-686-2234
Fax: 847-686-2251
Website: www.istss.org
E-mail: info@istss.org

National Headache Foundation (NHF)

820 N. Orleans
Ste. 201
Chicago, IL 60610-3131
Toll-Free: 888-NHF-5552
(888-643-5552)
Phone: 312-274-2650
Website: www.headaches.org
E-mail: info@headaches.org

Pediatric Brain Foundation (PBF)

2144 E. Republic Rd., Bldg. B.
Ste. 201
Springfield, MO 65804
Phone: 417-887-4242
Website: www.pediatricbrainfoun-dation.org
E-mail: info@pediatricbrainfoun-dation.org

Pediatric Brain Tumor Foundation (PBTF)

302 Ridgefield Ct.
Asheville, NC 28806
Toll-Free: 800-253-6530
Fax: 828-665-6894
Website: www.curethekids.org
E-mail: info@curethekids.org

Pulmonary Hypertension Association (PHA)

801 Roeder Rd.
Ste. 1000
Silver Spring, MD 20910
Toll-Free: 800-748-7274
Phone: 301-565-3004
Fax: 301-565-3994
Website: www.phassociation.org
E-mail: PHA@PHAssociation.org

INDEX

INDEX

Page numbers followed by 'n' indicate a footnote. Page numbers in *italics* indicate a table or illustration.

Administration for
  Community Living (ACL)
  contact 337
  publications
    disabilities 149n
    rehabilitation and life
      after traumatic brain
      injury (TBI) 253 n
    support services 301n
adrenaline, inner brain 7
aerobic exercise, returning to
  sports and activities 296
Agency for Healthcare
  Research and Quality
  (AHRQ)
  contact 337
  publication
    depression 103n
aggression
  domestic abuse 55
  epilepsy 134
  potential effects of TBI 29
  severe TBI 42
agitation
  concussion 39
  traumatic brain injury
    (TBI) 16
AHT *see* abusive head trauma
AIDS *see* acquired
  immunodeficiency
  syndrome
Air Carrier Access Act
  (ACAA), emotional support
  animals 164
AIS *see* Abbreviated Injury
  Scale
alcohol
  disability 142

alcohol, *continued*
  drug addiction 58
  epilepsy 135
  impaired driving 191
  mild TBI (mTBI) 87
  motorcycle safety 204
  pedestrian safety 215
  posttraumatic stress
    disorder (PTSD) 124
  substance abuse 61
  traumatic brain injury
    (TBI) 25
allergy and infectious diseases,
  clinical studies 321
altered consciousness,
  traumatic brain injury
  (TBI) 17
Alzheimer disease (AD)
  brain basics 10
  dementia and driving 226
  described 99
  potential effects of TBI 30
"Alzheimer Disease, Dementia,
  and Traumatic Brain Injury"
  (Omnigraphics) 99n
Alzheimer's Foundation of
  America (AFA), contact 339
amantadine, Parkinson disease
  (PD) 114
American Academy of
  Neurology (AAN), mild
  traumatic brain injury 22
American Brain Tumor
  Association (ABTA),
  contact 339
American Medical Society for
  Sports Medicine (AMSSM),
  mild traumatic brain injury 22

Index

349